ORIGINAL YOGA

ORIGINAL YOGA

Rediscovering Traditional Practices of Hatha Yoga

Richard Rosen

Illustrations by Evan Yee

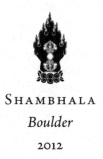

Shambhala
Boulder
2012

Shambhala Publications, Inc.
2129 13th Street
Boulder, Colorado 80302
www.shambhala.com

9 8 7 6 5 4

Printed in the United States of America

♾ This edition is printed on acid-free paper that meets the
American National Standards Institute z39.48 Standard.
♻ Shambhala Publications makes every effort to print on recycled paper.
For more information please visit www.shambhala.com.
Shambhala Publications is distributed worldwide by
Penguin Random House, Inc., and its subsidiaries.

Library of Congress Cataloging-in-Publication Data
Rosen, Richard.
Original yoga: rediscovering traditional practices of
Hatha yoga / Richard Rosen. — 1st ed.
p.   cm.
Includes bibliographical references and index.
ISBN 978-1-59030-813-4 (pbk.: alk. paper)
1. Hatha yoga. I. Title.
BL1238.56.H38R67 2012
613.7′046 — dc23
2011025817

Dedicated to my two best yoga friends

RY *and* TL

When it comes, you'll be dreaming
that you don't need to breathe;
that breathless silence is
the music of the dark
and it's part of the rhythm
to vanish like a spark.

—WISŁAWA SZYMBORSKA,
 "I'm Working on the World,"
 from *Calling Out to Yeti* (1957)

CONTENTS

ACKNOWLEDGMENTS

FIRST AND ALWAYS, thanks to Shambhala for giving me the opportunity to write this book, and to the two best editors in the world, Beth Frankl and Emily Bower, for all the invaluable help they gave me to make this book interesting and entertaining. I'd also like to thank my model, Chrisandra Fox, for her sterling performance of the poses in this book, and the artist, Evan Yee (whose father, I understand, is a yoga teacher), who turned my crude photos of Chrisandra into delicate line drawings. Finally, as always, thanks to all my teachers on whose shoulders I'm precariously perched, hoping to see a little bit farther into the distance. As usual with whatever I write, everything of value comes from them, while all the mistakes are mine alone.

ORIGINAL YOGA

INTRODUCTION

The Time Has Come
to Talk of Many Things

LET ME BEGIN by saying something about what I mean by "original yoga." Your immediate thought might be that what I'm presenting is a brand-new style of yoga, something original I've dreamed up that will join the ever-lengthening lineup of modern schools. But no, what's going on here is just the opposite. The original yoga I'll be talking about first is, as the book's subtitle suggests, traditional Hatha Yoga, which emerged around 900 C.E., give or take a couple of centuries in either direction. Of course, Hatha Yoga isn't the original yoga, the yoga school that preceded all others. That distinction formally belongs to the system outlined in Patanjali's *Yoga-Sutra*, compiled sometime between 200 B.C.E. and 200 C.E. But traditional Hatha Yoga does precede and is the "original" version of what we'll call modern Hatha Yoga, which began taking shape in the early decades of the twentieth century.

You may wonder why I'm making a distinction between traditional and modern Hatha Yoga. Isn't it all the same? Surprisingly, the answer is a resounding *no*. First of all, traditional Hatha Yoga, as it was practiced in India between the tenth and nineteenth centuries, certainly didn't stay the same all that time. If we compare the practice outlined in one of the school's granddaddy instruction manuals—the mid-fourteenth-century *Hatha-Yoga-Pradipika* (Light on Hatha Yoga)—with that of one

1

of its distant relatives — the late seventeenth-century *Gheranda-Samhita* (Gheranda's Compendium) — we find quite a few significant differences, not the least being that asana plays a much more important role in the latter book. But if we put the *Gheranda-Samhita* alongside one of its contemporaries, the *Shiva-Samhita* (Shiva's Compendium), we again find differences galore, such as the fact that asana is hardly mentioned at all in the latter. So first we need to recognize that the Hatha tradition isn't carved in stone; over its thousand-year run, it went through any number of changes, just as all of us do as we grow older. Our first order of business will be to look at this tradition as it's reflected in the three aforementioned books, taking the *Gheranda-Samhita* as our primary source backed up by the other two. I've chosen these three books because generally they're the easiest to come by in English translation. But be sure you understand that there are plenty of other books in the Hatha tradition, some a lot older than the *Hatha-Yoga-Pradipika,* some a bit younger than the *Gheranda-Samhita* and *Shiva-Samhita.*

Why do this at all, though? For the same reason many people look into their family's history: to better understand our present by delineating our past.

But what about the present? The changes the traditional practice went through over the centuries might be considered organic, common to any living organism's natural evolution. What happened to Hatha Yoga in the early years of the twentieth century, by contrast, happened virtually overnight and was totally "person-made," or artificial. The full story is too long to tell here and has already been masterfully recounted from slightly different perspectives by British researchers Elizabeth de Michelis in *A History of Modern Yoga* (Continuum, 2004) and Mark Singleton in *Yoga Body* (Oxford University Press, 2010; not to be confused with Judith Lasater's book *Yogabody*). Suffice it to say that by the end of the nineteenth century in India, Hatha had fallen on hard times and was on its last trembling leg. Several Indian teachers set out to save Hatha from oblivion; among them was Tirumular Krishnamacharya, whose work provided the impetus for three of our most popular and influential modern teachers: T. K. V. Desikachar (whose teaching was once known as Viniyoga, a term that has since been abandoned); the late K. Pattabhi Jois (who taught Ashtanga-Vinyasa Yoga); and B. K. S. Iyengar, who (though he often adamantly insists there's no such thing) created Iyengar Yoga. And save Hatha the teachers did. You may have heard or read somewhere that yoga is five thousand years old, a number that's continually cited by people who should know better, since there's not a shred of concrete evidence to back it up. What we do know for certain is that the yoga we practice in the West is no more than one hundred years old. Our Indian teachers took what was once the province of a relatively small, loose-knit, mostly male ascetic community that was resolutely living on the fringes of respectable Indian society and transformed it into a worldwide mass movement open to anyone of any age, gender, or physical condition. This is the second meaning of *original yoga,* the yoga that's "original" to the twentieth century, or what we call modern Hatha Yoga.

What is modern yoga all about? Traditional Hatha Yoga is what might be called a "full-time job"—time-consuming, strenuous, physically dangerous, and morally objectionable to mainstream standards in more ways than one. If the practice was to appeal to a popular audience, corners had to be cut so that the average householder-practitioner could fit a practice into her busy schedule, and dangerous or objectionable exercises had to be modified or excised altogether. When the dust of renovation settled, there really wasn't much left to do, so exercises were imported from outside sources—Indian wrestling and Western gymnastics—to beef up the practice. They were given Sanskrit names to make them seem "yogic"; in this way, modern Hatha Yoga became asana-centric, or more precisely, it became equated with asana. In fact, most "yoga" classes (including those at my studio in Oakland), books, and videos nowadays are "asana" classes, books, and videos. I'm not here to criticize this development, as many traditionalists do; I actually believe that the modern "asana-ization" of Hatha Yoga was a good thing, a way to draw hyper, body-image-conscious Westerners into the fold and get them hooked. According to both the *Hatha-Yoga-Pradipika* and *Gheranda-Samhita,* the first stage of traditional Hatha Yoga isn't the behavioral injunctions—the *yamas* and *niyamas,* as it is in Patanjali's yoga—but asana. What we Westerners have been doing for the last sixty or so years is just that, practicing the first traditional Hatha stage, preparing ourselves for . . . what?

This what brings us to the third meaning of original yoga. *Original* can also mean "showing a marked departure from previous practice," so just as modern Hatha was a marked departure from its traditional predecessor, so the practice presented in this book is a marked departure from modern Hatha Yoga. It's not, mind you, original in the sense of something new; rather, it's original because the practice largely returns to the tradition. After several years of studying the old books, I realized that in the Indian teachers' run-up to modern Hatha, a few babies were tossed out with the bathwater, leaving gaping holes in our practice that rendered it ineffective in many ways, especially spiritually. I dug mostly into the *Gheranda-Samhita* and *Hatha-Yoga-Pradipika*—the *Shiva-Samhita* is largely philosophical, while its two companions basically ignore philosophy and focus on practical matters—and came out with a good many traditional exercises that are still appropriate for nonspecialist practitioners. Let me be clear: I'm not advocating a return to the old ways. Traditional Hatha Yoga, at least in this country, is a thing of the past, but certain traditional practices can still have a powerful transformative effect. What I imagine doing is paradoxically taking a step back to take a step forward.

But this step forward is, as the old saying goes, the beginning of a thousand-mile journey. Yoga was born, nurtured, and cultivated in India, but it's been passed along to the West like the baton in a relay race. For all intents and purposes, over the last six decades, we've refined the original foundation practice—asana—far beyond the wildest imaginings of the old yogis. But although we are asana adults, the rest of our practice is still in its infancy. So now it's time to turn our attention to other matters, using the traditional practice as our model but shaping the practice to suit Western needs.

1

TRADITIONAL HATHA YOGA

HATHA · violence, force; obstinacy,
pertinacity; absolute or inevitable necessity
(as the cause of all existence and activity)

WHAT IS HATHA YOGA?

I sometimes teach a course on the philosophy of traditional Hatha Yoga, since the proponents of this school agreed with the French philosopher Blaise Pascal, who said, "To have no time for philosophy is to be a true philosopher." I always like to begin, as I'm doing now, with a few basic definitions, just to make sure everyone in the room is on the same page. Naturally the opening question is, what do we mean by *yoga*? Most students answer this query with a single word like *union* or *yoking* (the latter is cognate with *yoga,* the former isn't), which is a perfectly good half-answer but not the whole one. To get that, we have to go back a few thousand years when, once upon a time, in a galaxy halfway around the world, the Sanskrit word *yoga* referred in general to the yoking of animals to a cart, particularly warhorses to a chariot. These equines were what we would call "hyper" and at best uncooperative—something like a certain teenager of my acquaintance—when it came to being told what to do and harnessed to a chariot. The person in charge of the yoking, the charioteer (who also drove the vehicle while his rider, the warrior, wreaked havoc on their enemies) needed special training to manage his job efficiently and effectively and, just as important, to avoid getting trampled in the process. To achieve his goal, which was union or yoking, he needed a time-tested method, no doubt learned at the knee of a more experienced mentor. So the word *yoga* has two essential meanings that go together like a horse and carriage. As the Sanskrit dictionary defines it, yoga is both "the act of yoking, joining, attaching, harnessing, putting to (of horses)," and "a means, expedient, device, way, manner, method." This draws a vivid analogy between the charioteer and the yoga practitioner. Like the former, the latter is dealing with an unruly "beast" — his own consciousness, which he must learn to handle with the assistance of appropriate means or techniques, so that his embodied or "living self" (*jiva atman*) can be yoked (or reyoked) with its source, the "great self" (*parama atman*). We can say then, to fill in the other half of our definition, that *yoga* properly means "union-method."

So far, so good, but we're not quite done yet. Next we need to ask, what do we mean by *hatha*? It's interesting that the answer I get to this question is almost invariably "sun-moon," which again isn't exactly wrong, but it's not exactly right either. At least it's not the answer this trick question is looking for. Many words in the yoga lexicon have both an "outer" and an "inner" meaning: the former is literal, the dictionary definition; the latter is figurative, assigned to the word by the tradition to drive home some telling point about the person or practice referred to, but otherwise an etymological fabrication. This is typically done by dividing the word into its constituent syllables and assigning a usually (but not always) arbitrary definition to each; when combined, they yield a meaning that's greater than the sum of the word's parts. In the case of *hatha, ha* is taken to mean "sun" (which it doesn't) and *tha* to mean "moon" (which it does in some contexts). These two celestial bodies represent our primary psychoenergetic principles, what Patanjali termed the "pairs of opposites" (*dvandva*; literally "two-two"), though just as accurately and more appropriately for Hatha Yoga, they might be called the "pairs of complements." These energies — signified variously as hot and cold, light and dark, male and female — are the motivating forces in our lives, constantly pushing and pulling us back and forth in a lifelong tug-of-war, measuring out the years of our current incarnation. In Patanjali's yoga, these pairs are obstacles to liberation and so are ultimately transcended, that is, left behind when the eternal, static self frees itself from the trammels of its mistaken identification with ephemeral, changeable matter. But in Hatha Yoga, the pairs are accepted as integral to our identity and so are embraced by the practice. The fragmented energies are brought together at the "middle" of our being, and the body is thereby transformed to serve as a suitable vehicle for our liberation.

So if "sun-moon" is the inner meaning of *hatha,* what's the outer meaning? I always enjoy the moment in class (less exciting in a book) when I dramatically reveal that *hatha* literally means "force" or "violence." The audience usually reacts to this with either wide-eyed disbelief or narrow-eyed skepticism. "How could that be?" I can almost hear them saying to themselves. "Isn't yoga well known for its let-go attitude and emphasis on *nonviolence?*" It does seem like a contradiction, but it tells us that there is indeed a disconnect between traditional Hatha Yoga and its modern counterpart. The practice is commonly presented nowadays as a way to relax and release the symptoms of stress, but it's a "part-time job" for most students, a small part of their lives, no matter how much it nourishes them. But for old-timers, yoga was a full-time job; it was serious business pursued with "great effort" (*bahu yatna*), both physical and psychological, to relieve the source of all stress, which is ignorance (*avidya*) of the authentic self.

Now we have enough background information to answer the $64,000 Question: what do we mean by *Hatha Yoga?* The straightforward reply is the "forceful union-method," though we have to be cautious about how we interpret *forceful.* To avoid a potentially injurious misunderstanding, it's probably best qualified with *appropriate,* or as the police sometimes say, *necessary.* So in Hatha Yoga, we're applying appropriate force, first, to transform our physical body to serve as a suitable vehicle for liberation and, second, to (re-)connect and (re-)integrate our fragmented energies and realize our essential wholeness. However this is not the only way to interpret *Hatha Yoga.* Yoga scholar Georg Feuerstein suggests an alternative: the "yoga of the force." What does this mean? The "force" here isn't what Luke Skywalker put to good use in *Star Wars;* it is the "mysterious *kundalini,*" or as in the title of the classic study by John Woodroffe, the "serpent power." Literally the "coiled one," *kundalini* is best thought of for the time being as our dormant spiritual potential, the awakening and fulfillment of which is a central concern in Hatha Yoga. In either case, the practice involves some measure of force, whether we exert that force on ourselves in the service of transformation or transform ourselves through the power of a force (which can be unleashed by appropriately forceful means) that is considered our most precious possession.

These somewhat long-winded definitions have two purposes: one, to make sure, just as I do in my courses, that we share an understanding of two basic terms as a starting point for our study; and two, as a lead-in to the idea behind this book. Just as there are inner and outer definitions of certain key yoga words, so too there are inner and outer "stories" about Hatha Yoga. The outer story is right now being written by groundbreaking yoga scholars and historians (see *The Yoga Upanishads* in appendix 2). These writers give us the dictionary definition of Hatha Yoga, with accounts of its origins and earliest influences, its semilegendary founders and lineage teachers, its evolution over ten centuries, its gradual fall from grace to near extinction in the late nineteenth century, and its floor-to-ceiling renovation and grand reopening in the early decades of the twentieth century.

But there's also the inner story of Hatha Yoga. Not found in any dictionary, it has been passed along through at least forty generations of yogis both orally and in mostly obscure and arcane books, some of which have found their way into English. What are we to make of these inner stories from unknown or long-forgotten practitioners? We often scan them from our lofty, bird's-eye, twenty-first-century perspective with either skepticism or indulgence, as if they were produced by charlatans who wanted to pull the wool over our eyes for their own nefarious purposes or by overly imaginative children. We readily accept (or at least don't readily dismiss) the outer story, which comforts and reassures us with its painstaking research, literate style, and meticulous footnotes. But the inner story, which reads more like an outlandish fantasy, makes twenty-first-century, rational-minded people uncomfortable. What are we to make of completely serious reports of divine intercessions and miraculous births; seemingly simple exercises leading to superhuman powers; or wrinkled graybeards turning into beautiful youths or extending their years beyond those of Methuselah, even beyond the dissolution of the entire universe?

One obvious explanation—not too popular in the yoga community—is that these men were seriously deluded, that many of their extreme breathing or meditation exercises overloaded their brain circuitry
and blew out more than a few neural fuses in the process. Another explanation—more acceptable and probable—is that these same exercises
altered their view of the consensus reality of their time and, like Dorothy
and Toto, they were lifted out of Kansas and deposited in some magical
realm where scarecrows talked and monkeys flew. You might have had an
inkling of what it's like in the yoga version of Oz in your own yoga career.
When leaving an especially rousing class, have you ever felt that you were
"flying"? Or that somehow you were a different person than the one who
walked in at the start of class? That you felt more youthful, energetic,
as if you would live forever? Take these feelings, generated from a mere
sixty- or ninety-minute class, and then magnify them a hundred times;
you might get a taste of what the ancient yogis were talking about.

So what these men were talking about—and, more important, what
practices led them to their (re-)vision of the world—is one good way
to describe the subject of this book. To step into the old yogis' shoes
and set off on a jaunt through their world, we'll take along a bag full of
guidebooks, three of which are considered by most experts to be the
foundations of traditional Hatha Yoga, as already noted in the Introduction. The oldest of the trio is the *Hatha-Yoga-Pradipika,* which we can
now properly translate as "Light on the Forceful Union-Method." We
also previewed the other two Baedekers, the contemporaneous *Shiva-
Samhita* and *Gheranda-Samhita,* the latter supplying the bulk of material for this book. Now that we've defined what we mean by the words
yoga and *hatha,* it's time to relate what the teaching of Hatha Yoga
is about.

GHERANDA AND CHANDA

The *Gheranda-Samhita* is set within the framework of a conversation between the guru Gheranda and Chanda, a wandering ascetic. Dialogue is a
common literary device in these old books to get the ball rolling, though
in truth there isn't much of a dialogue here. After asking Gheranda to

teach him yoga, Chanda pretty much disappears into the background, and Gheranda does the lion's share of the talking. Still, the device allows the reader to identify vicariously with the pupil, giving a feel for what it might be like to sit face-to-face with a guru and hear his teaching directly.

LITTLE LAMP: SALUTATION

shri adinathaya namo'sthu tasmai yenopadishta hathayogavidya |
vibhrajate pronnatarajayogamarodumichchhoradhirohiniva ||

"Prosperity, welfare, good fortune, success, auspiciousness; power, might, majesty" (*shri*)! We salute the "first lord" (*adi natha*, i.e., Shiva) who "taught, prescribed, commanded" (*upadishta*) the wisdom (*vidya*) of Hatha Yoga. It's the "ladder, flight of steps" (*adhirohin*) we can climb to Royal Yoga (*Raja Yoga*).

— Opening salutation in the *Hatha-Yoga-Pradipika*

A D I · beginning, commencement; a firstling, first fruits
N A T H A · protector, patron, possessor, owner, lord; a rope passed through the nose of a draft ox
S H I V A · "in whom all things lie"; perhaps connected with *shvi*, "to swell"; auspicious, propitious, gracious, kind, happy, fortunate; liberation; "auspicious one"

Often the old Hatha books begin with a nod to a sage or deity, typically Shiva, as the source of the Hatha teaching. The opening verse of the *Hatha-Yoga-Pradipika* pays homage to Shiva as the "first lord," which may be understood in a couple of ways. Shiva is, for the yogis, the reigning god of all the gods, the first among equals. But he's also first in the lineage of Hatha Yoga, the source of all Hatha wisdom (*vidya*). *Natha* is usually rendered as "lord," but notice in the preceding translation that it also means "protector." Hatha Yoga then is a "return to the source" of power, a reconnection with our authentic self. (Of course, the separation is only apparent, not real. Transcendent unity can never be truly broken). As we look for the source, the source is looking for us, and it draws us to itself. Once we realize our self as source, then it's incumbent on us to also become "patrons," to assist others to find their way home. Notice that a *natha* is also a kind of leash, and we are forever joined to the source by the source itself. Svatmarama tells us (*Hatha-Yoga-Pradipika* 4.54ff.) to take refuge (*ashrita*) in this "motionless, immovable, fixed, steady, invariable, unchangeable" (*nishchala*) source.

The word *guru* entered everyday English around the middle of the last century. We use it willy-nilly to refer to a mentor or an expert in, say, economics or politics. But in the yoga tradition, the word is applied narrowly to a self-realized spiritual preceptor who, because of his or her great spiritual achievement, is treated with the utmost respect and reverence. We see this in the way Chanda modestly approaches Gheranda, bowing in obeisance and addressing him as "Yoga Master" (*yogesha*) and "Yoga Lord" (*yogeshvara*). *Guru*, like *hatha*, has both an outer and an inner meaning. Literally it means "weighty" or "heavy" (*guru* is a distant relative of the Latin *gravis*, or "heavy," from which we get "gravity"). The suggestion is that such a teacher is plump or pregnant with divine wisdom. Its inner meaning is derived from its two syllables, as the *Guru-Gita* (33) explains: "The syllable *gu* is the darkness, and the syllable *ru* is said to be light. There is no doubt that the Guru is indeed the Supreme Knowledge that dispels (the darkness of) ignorance."

In the old days, the only way you could learn yoga was through initiation by a guru. There were no drop-ins back then, and students were chosen with care only after they had demonstrated their worthiness and commitment. So the guru was literally all-powerful, revered as mother, father, and God himself; his words, unlike those of the average person, were charged with transformative power. Nowadays, we can buy a copy of the exchange between Gheranda and Chanda for a few dollars on Amazon.com. Because it's so easily and cheaply acquired, we might tend to take for granted and undervalue the teaching once thought to be priceless. Like Matsyendra in the great fish's belly (see pages 141–42), we're about to be privy to normally hard-won information. Thus, we should heed Gheranda's advice to Chanda as he launches into his teaching, which is, "Listen carefully, attentively to what I'm about to say. Apply your mind only to my words" (*savadhano'vadharaya*).

LITTLE LAMP: THE MODERN INDIAN
GURU ARCHETYPE

We all have an image of the wise, stern, but compassionate Indian guru. If we look carefully at the biographies of our modern gurus, can we draw a picture of what the typical "heavy one" may look like? The following portrait is based on the life stories of Swami Rama Tirtha, Paramahamsa Yogananda, Shri Yogendra, Jiddu Krishnamurti, Swami Prabhavananda, Swami Omkar, Tirumular Krishnamcharya, B. K. S. Iyengar, K. Pattabhi Jois, Maharishi Mahesh Yogi, Swami Muktananda, Swami Sivananda, Swami Prabhupada, Swami Rama, Swami Vivekananda, Yogi Bhajan, Amrit Desai, Baba Premananda Bharati, Bhagwan Shri Rajneesh, Swami Satchidananda.

- The future guru is always male. His economic class varies; many come from the upper-middle class, while others grow up in relative poverty (though most are typically born to a Brahmin family). He's often born at some astrologically propitious time, in a spiritually significant place, or during a spiritually significant festival.
- An astrologer/spiritual master predicts great things for him.
- He's often unusually smart for his age (or at least reported to be by his admittedly biased biographers), sometimes debating with adults, exhibiting psychic powers or visions, or displaying spiritual inclinations or flashes of illumination. He also sometimes shows heartwarming compassion for the poor (and untouchables), animals, and so forth.
- He often has a traditional spiritual upbringing, sometimes taught by his father from spiritual texts (like the *Rigveda*) in Sanskrit. His mother is usually deeply religious.
- He's often an outstanding student and educated at a Western-style school (sometimes run by Christians), though sometimes he's a poor student, despite an expensive Western education (as in the case of Krishnamurti). He also displays other remarkable talents or gifts (in areas such as singing, acting, athletic ability, or writing).
- As a result of his superior intellectual and artistic abilities, family and friends widely agree that he's destined for a successful career in

the world (such as a mathematics or philosophy professor, a doctor, or an engineer), though sometimes he may struggle financially.

- Sometimes a parent dies when the boy is young or his wife dies early in their marriage, which may precipitate a spiritual search (detailed later in this list).
- He may work at some high-paying job, but he is ultimately unsatisfied by material life, and his spiritual longings become overpowering.
- He almost always has a guru (almost always male), and usually this is his guru for life. He often meets the guru in a chance encounter. He may immediately recognize and accept his guru, or he may go through a difficult period of doubt before committing. The initiation is usually a deeply transformative experience.
- Usually, he's completely dedicated to his guru, but sometimes the relationship is rocky (as with Krishnamacharya and Iyengar; the latter seems to be an exception to most of these rules).
- The guru performs "miracles" (such as healing the sick and lame, predicting the future, and materializing objects out of thin air).
- There's often a period of wandering in the wilderness (for months or even years), whether in self-reflection (sometimes after a death in the family); while following his guru; or if he hasn't yet found him, in search of his true guru (especially in the Himalayas but sometimes throughout India).
- Occasionally he has progressive ideas for his time and place (for example, favoring female education or rejecting caste distinctions), though he can also be a strict traditionalist.
- He often has a wealthy patron (such as a successful businessman or royalty).
- He leaves India for the West (with the exceptions of Krishnamacharya and Sivananda) for different reasons. He may be sent on a mission by his guru to spread Hindu "gospel" to the world; he may raise money for social causes; or he may heed a call from within.
- His message is often well received in the West. He attracts well-to-do supporters who give him money and property, and he sometimes amasses a personal fortune.

- He establishes an ashram, organization, or institute (usually in a large city or highly desirable locale) that either grows and spreads across the country or dies out after he leaves the country.
- Sometimes he develops an innovative practice that he synthesizes from various existing practices, though he often tries to associate his invention with traditional teachings.
- If he returns to India, he's often welcomed as a hero.
- He often undergoes a miraculous death (which is usually not described as "dying" but as entering *maha samadhi,* or "leaving his body," as if it were intentional). Sometimes something miraculous happens after his death (for example, his body doesn't decay).

I have an Indian miniature hanging on my office wall that I bought many years ago in New Delhi. It shows an aged, white-bearded gentleman squatting on a tiger-skin rug (a typical "sticky mat" for devotees of Shiva) in front of a small cottage, one long string of beads draped around his neck and another over his left arm. Kneeling deferentially beside him is a well-dressed young man wearing a jaunty, feathered turban and holding out a ring for the old man's acceptance. It doesn't take much imagination to figure out the story being told by this painting. The elder is surely a guru of weighty wisdom, both mundane and spiritual; the former is suggested by a pair of books lying on the ground by his feet and the latter by a ceremonial white conch shell lying next to the books. The young man is a petitioner and his ring an offering — a down payment, as it were, for the guru's teaching. The guru regards the young man and the ring dispassionately through half-shuttered eyes, his arms crossed in front of his chest, not making the slightest move to reach out for the ring. It's apparent that he isn't much interested in the ring and that the young man needs a better plan of action if he wants an education.

We can assume our classroom, with Gheranda as the headmaster, is much like the one in my painting. The story begins, as so many fairy tales do, *ekada* (which can be rendered "one day," "once," or as I prefer, "once upon a time") Chanda paid a visit to Gheranda at his cottage. The old books were generally specific about what this residence should look like and where it should be located (*Hatha-Yoga-Pradipika* 1.12–14 and

Gheranda-Samhita 5.4–7). Anonymous/Gheranda calls it a *kutira,* Svat-marama a *matha;* both of these terms mean "hut" or "cottage," though *matha* refers specifically to the "retired hut (or cell) of an ascetic." I point out this usage because a few verses earlier Svatmarama declares that Hatha Yoga itself is a *matha.* I can't say if he was intentionally drawing a parallel here or not, but we might conclude that just as Gheranda's cottage physically sheltered him from the elements, so Hatha Yoga figuratively sheltered him from sorrow and pain (for pain, Svatmarama uses the word *tapas,* meaning "consuming heat" or "causing pain or trouble").

LITTLE LAMP: WHY ANONYMOUS/GHERANDA?

It's been said (and I've not been able to find the source of this quote) that even authors who write in praise of humility take care to put their names on the title page. This is undoubtably true about modern authors, including myself, but it isn't at all the case when we consider the old yogis and their writing. Isaac Newton once said, "If I have seen further it is only by standing on the shoulders of giants," and this is exactly what many old yogi writers believed. The considered their work to be the product of a group effort reaching back through the centuries, and so often declined to take credit for it. Instead they attributed their writing to someone else, either another yogi or a deity. This applies to two of our three main books. While we know the author of the *Hatha-Yoga-Pradipika,* the authors of the *Gheranda-Samhita* and *Shiva-Samhita* are unknown, either because their names were lost over the last three or four centuries, or because their names were, for reasons known only to them, never given.

The cottage is described as small and windowless, its walls plastered with cow dung (apparently an excellent insulator and mosquito repellent), its yard ideally including an arbor, a well, and of course a meditation platform. This latter is supposed to be high enough to raise the yogi off the ground and out of the way of creepy things, but not so high that a misstep would send him tumbling disastrously heels over head. By tradition, it's covered with kusha grass, a deer or tiger skin (symbol of primal energy), or a blanket. Kusha grass, sacred to the Hindus, was used to cover ceremonial altars well back into Vedic times, at least two thousand years earlier. This suggests that the platform is akin to an altar, where instead of clarified butter the yogi offers his own self-ignorance as a sacrifice. Usually called an *asana*, Svatmarama names the platform a *vedi*, meaning "pedestal, stand, bench." Again, I can't say if this was intentional or not, but *vedi* also refers both to a "wise man" and the Vedic altar, believed to be "earth's most central station" (*Rig Veda* 10.1.a6), where the gods sat while attending the ceremony.

We usually picture our gurus living a secluded life in the wilds, high on a mountaintop or deep in some forest clearing. But Svatmarama and Gheranda agree that a yogi's cottage should be situated somewhere between the Outback and downtown Manhattan: far enough away from town so the yogi can avoid the distractions of noise and pollution and entanglements with people, but at the same time close enough to a decent-sized population center so he can benefit from its relatively ready and reliable availability of sustenance. The local town should be "good for begging" (*su bhikhsa*). But not only the immediate vicinity needs to be conducive to the yogi's practice: the country he lives in should be well-governed, virtuous (*dharmika*, meaning "righteous, pious") and free of "national commotions."

Now we can ask, who was Gheranda? It's impossible to say with any certainty, since there's no Facebook-like profile of him anywhere in the *Gheranda-Samhita* or, for that matter, anywhere in the Hatha Yoga tradition that I can find. Was he an actual person or a fictional mouthpiece dreamed up by the real author? At least one modern scholar seems confidant of the former: in his classic 1938 study *Gorakhnath and the Kanphata Yogis*, George Weston Briggs stated without qualification that Gheranda was a "Vaishnavite of Bengal"[1]; in plain English, he was a devotee of the deity Vishnu living in eastern India (either that or what is now Bangladesh, which was once a part of India). Is there any evidence to support this claim in the book? There's one verse near the end of the story (*Gheranda-Samhita* 7.18, cf. 5.77) extolling Vishnu, which sounds like it issues from a true believer. Vishnu, it says, can be found in water (*jala*), in earth (*sthala*), on the summit of mountains (*parvata mastaka*); in short, the entire universe (*jagat*) is made of Vishnu. Of course, this doesn't prove the historicity of Gheranda himself, only that the author of the book was a Vaishnava (or had Vaishnava sympathies). As if covering all the deity bases, the next verse (*Gheranda-Samhita* 7.19) assures us that all the creatures of the earth and skies, all the plants, and the mountains are Brahma; a little further along (*Gheranda-Samhita* 7.22), the author credits his teaching to Shiva.

Now what about Chanda? His name means "fierce, passionate," which we can assume betokens his passion for yoga and his ferocity in pursuing liberation. The appellation Skull Bearer (*kapalika*) tells us he was a member of an infamous ascetic sect with associations to Hatha Yoga. Surviving accounts of the Kapalikas condemn their appearance and behavior, though such accounts were written primarily by their legions of mainstream detractors (Kapalikas not surprisingly didn't leave behind much of a written record). We can expect that these diatribes were exaggerated to some degree, though it's obvious that the sect members encouraged—maybe even relished—these negative reactions by wandering the countryside naked, their long hair piled atop their heads, their bodies smeared with funeral ashes, menacingly armed with a trident or iron-tipped bamboo staff, using a hollow cranium for a begging bowl . . . you get the picture.

LITTLE LAMP: SKULL BEARER (KAPALIKA)

Why did Chandra carry around a skull? The backstory to this has several different versions, the common element among them being an unfortunate incident involving Brahma and Shiva. One version describes an argument between the two over who's more supreme, a battle of egos that seems rather inappropriate for a pair of deities. Another version has Brahma insulting Shiva, and a third has Shiva protecting the honor of a young woman pursued by Brahma. Whatever the case, all the stories agree that because of what transpired, Shiva assaulted Brahma and lopped off one of his five heads with the tip of the fingernail of Shiva's left thumb. This might not seem like much to us (after all, Brahma had four more heads), but to the Hindus of the time it was a heinous crime, "brahma killing" (*brahma hatya*), the worst kind of karma imaginable. Brahma cursed Shiva (or Shiva's agent Bhairava) to wander the earth as both a punishment and penance, begging for his livelihood with a skull as his begging bowl. The Kapalikas, great admirers of Shiva, emulated him and, because they were innocent yet underwent punishment and did penance, generating a vast store of good karma that they hoped would make them godly like Shiva.

The Kapalikas had largely disappeared in India by the fourtheenth century, so we might wonder about Chanda's presence in a tale written, as experts assure us, some 350 to 400 years later. Perhaps Anonymous/ Gheranda was harking back to an earlier time to make it appear that his compendium was older than it actually was. It's well known that traditional Indians' esteem for a book or teaching increases proportionally with its age: the older the book, the more they venerate it. That's why we so frequently hear or read that yoga is five thousand years old, an impressive number unsubstantiated by any concrete evidence. Another possibility is that Anonymous/Gheranda wanted a figure who was widely recognized as a hard-core outsider, someone known to break all the rules and flaunt authority, so that Chanda's deference to Gheranda would seal the latter's cachet as a spiritual heavy hitter. But whatever the reason for Chanda's presence, and despite the Kapalikas' collective bad-boy reputation, Gheranda accepts him as a student without hesitation. The guru greets him with the honorific *sadhu* (spoken not once, but twice for emphasis), literally "kind, willing, obedient; successful, effective, peaceful, secure; powerful, excellent; good, virtuous, honorable, righteous."

But he's not done yet. In the next breath (*Gheranda-Samhita* 1.3), Gheranda praises Chanda as "mighty arms" (*maha baho*). When I first read this, it struck me as odd that the sage would use this epithet for the Skull Bearer. Certainly we aren't meant to picture Chanda as some kind of seventeenth-century Conan the Barbarian. Then I remembered that the charioteer Krishna used the same nickname (one among many) for the warrior Arjuna in the *Bhagavad-Gita* (2.68). Again, I can't say if this was intentional, but it's possible that Anonymous/Gheranda was drawing a parallel between our two humble yogis and the dynamic duo of the *Gita*. If this is something more than my overheated imagination, then our two obscure yogis and this little prelude to the teaching take on mythic dimensions. Gheranda is revealed as Krishna, the embodiment of the great self (Vishnu), while mighty-armed Chandra becomes Arjuna, the living self (*jiva atman*), a spark of the great self and representative of all humanity. Lastly though, as if to bring the proceedings back to earth in preparation for the upcoming lessons and show his own human, compassionate side, Gheranda agrees to deliver the goods and lovingly calls Chanda "my dear child" (*vatsa*).

LITTLE LAMP: *GRIHASTHA* ("HOUSEHOLDER")

It's all well and good to be a yogi as a confirmed ascetic, when your only responsibility all day long is to yourself and your practice, but what about someone with a day job, a family, and a mortgage? Could a householder practice yoga too? Gheranda doesn't say, but Anonymous/Shiva does: as long as such a person conducts his or her business without "attachment" (*raga*), even living in a house filled with children (*putra*) and a wife (*dara*) or husband, a householder can achieve success (*siddhi*). And, Anonymous/Shiva concludes, have a "good time" (*krida*).

GHERANDA'S TEACHING

So what is the substance of Gheranda's teaching? Actually, after Chanda's big buildup, his obsequious Yoga Master this and Yoga Lord that, Gheranda's presentation is somewhat disappointing. Old yoga hands will recognize his worldview as standard fare and no doubt second the pull-no-punches opinion of the *Encyclopedia of Indian Philosophies*: "The text is largely a Hatha Yoga manual of practice and contains almost nothing of any philosophical importance."[2] It seems that by the time the *Gheranda-Samhita* was composed, much of Hatha Yoga's early in-your-face, I'll-do-it-my-way attitude had been replaced by a more conciliatory tone to make it more acceptable to the mainstream. If we want a full picture of the ideas that provided a framework for Hatha practice, we'll need to supplement Gheranda with material from Svatmarama and Anonymous/Shiva.

Though he doesn't elaborate on it much, Gheranda provides a kind of outline of his teaching at the outset. For convenience, we can call the points he emphasizes the Four Fs (based on the English translation of the Sanskrit), which team up naturally in opposing pairs:

- Fetter (*pasha;* "snare, trap, noose") and foe (*ripu;* "cheat, rogue") on one side
- Force (*bala;* "power, might") and friend (*bandhu;* "kinsman") on the other side

It's easy now to paint this in by the numbers, though we have to be careful of our colors. The foe in Gheranda's mind is the *ahamkara,* literally the "I-maker" or what we call the ego, which fetters or binds us to an illusion (*maya*) about ourselves and the world, the cause of our unremitting existential sorrow (which Svatmarama calls *tapas*). It's true that the ego is a limiting factor in space and time, but that's its job—to create boundaries. It's not fair to point a finger at the ego as the source of our difficulty. Rather, the problem is our understandable but mistaken identification with and belief in the ego as our true self, which Gheranda describes near the end of the book as pure consciousness (*chaitanya*) that is nondual (*advaita;* literally "not-two," figuratively "having no duplicate, peerless, sole, unique; the ultimate truth"), eternal (*shashvata;* "perpetual, all"), and supreme (*para*).

We should be sure not to demonize the ego as the enemy but practice to relegate it to its proper place and role in the overall ecology of our consciousness. If we fail to do this, Gheranda warns, we're doomed to wander through life aimlessly (*bhrama*), asleep at the wheel and repeating the same mistaken, often self-destructive behaviors over and over. He uses the image of the waterwheel going around and around, its buckets filling and emptying ceaselessly. (This is not as powerful an image today as it was in the seventeenth century. We might respond more readily to the image of an escalator moving continuously or a bicycle chain going around.)

What do we need to do to break this painful cycle? Gheranda advises us to seek help from our best friend (*bandhu*)—knowledge (*jnana*). Notice the word Gheranda uses here: translating *jnana* as "knowledge" isn't wrong, but it's slightly misleading because we English speakers immediately associate the word only with book learning or erudition, exactly the kind of knowledge for which many of our so-called gurus are prized. Gheranda doesn't discount such worldly knowledge, but he wants us to realize that *jnana* has a further denotation that's often termed — as my Sanskrit dictionary phrases it, though I don't particularly like it — "higher knowledge." Actually, *jnana* is cognate with a little-used English word, *gnosis* (both stem from the verb *jna*, "to know"), that expresses this second meaning perfectly. As my dictionary defines it, *gnosis* is the "intuitive apprehension of spiritual truths, an esoteric form of knowledge," which is exactly the *bandhu* to which Gheranda is referring. And just how do we acquire this gnosis? By the transformative power, strength, might, and vigor (*bala*) generated by the practice of yoga, of course.

After all this, we must ask, to what conclusion is all this leading? Gheranda draws a parallel between the two levels of *jnana*: just as studying the alphabet (*varna*) eventually leads to our ability to read and understand the scriptures (*shashtras*), so does our study of yoga lead to direct insight into the truth (*tattva*) about our self. Here Gheranda uses the word *tattva*, which is *guru* with meaning: "true or real state, truth, reality; the essence or substance of anything; knowledge of truth, thorough knowledge, insight into . . . true principles." *Tattva*, as the yogis parse it, is composed of two words: *tad* ("that," implying the great self or Brahman), and *tvam* ("you," implying the embodied self); taken together, they yield what's called the great assertion (*maha vakya*), or *tad tvam*, "that [is] you." We might call this the verbal string around the finger, a reminder of something we've forgotten but need to remember above all else.

THE YOGA OF THE POT (*GHATASTHA YOGA*)

So how do we reach the *tattva*? I'm sure you can easily guess the answer: according to Svatmarama (*Hatha-Yoga-Pradipika* 1.1), by climbing the ladder (*adirohana*) provided by Hatha Yoga. Incidentally, something he writes in this verse has led to a good deal of confusion. Instead of naming *tattva* as the goal of practice, Svatmarama uses the phrase *raja yoga* ("royal union-method"), which is commonly applied to Patanjali's eight-limb system. A number of modern teachers, who might not have read the *Hatha-Yoga-Pradipika* as closely as they could have, have mistakenly concluded that Hatha Yoga is a mere physical preparation for Patanjali's yoga. The next time someone makes this claim in your presence, kindly refer them to *Hatha-Yoga-Pradipika* 4.4 (or *Gheranda-Samhita* 7.17), where Svatmarama explicitly states that Raja Yoga is a synonym for *samadhi*.

LITTLE LAMP: *SAMADHI*

SAMADHI · putting together, joining or combining with; union, a whole, an aggregate; completion, accomplishment, conclusion; setting to rights, adjustment, settlement; justification of a statement, proof; bringing into harmony, agreement, assent; intense application or fixing the mind on, intentness, attention; concentration of the thoughts, profound or abstract meditation, intense contemplation of any particular object (so as to identify the contemplator with the object being meditated on; the eighth and last stage of yoga); intense absorption, a kind of trance

We'll run across this word often in the sourcebooks, so what is *samadhi*? It is, of course, the eighth limb of Patanjali's eight-limb yoga, the last before the practitioner achieves total release or "isolation" (*kaivalya*). In Hatha Yoga, *samadhi* seems to indicate the condition of ultimate release itself.

Oddly enough, or maybe interestingly enough, Gheranda doesn't call his version of Hatha Yoga "Hatha Yoga." Rather, he names it Ghatastha Yoga (*Gheranda-Samhita* 1.2), the "union-method of the pot" (*ghata*). Pot? None of my *Gheranda-Samhita* source translators literally translate *ghata* as "pot," choosing instead to leave it unhelpfully untranslated or render it as what they believe Gheranda was implying by the image, something like "body," "physical body," or "physiological body." There's nothing terribly wrong with these translations, but none of them quite accurately conveys the sense of what Gheranda intends by "pot." The image may be a remnant of the influence of Hindu alchemy on proto–Hatha Yoga. Here the yogi is compared to the alchemist: just as the latter conducted his transformative experiments in a pot, the former does the same in his body. It's also possible that the pot (*kumbha*) may have ritual associations or that it symbolizes the "womb, the generative power," or the "Divine in general" as a container of "life, sustenance, and fertility."[3]

The problem with using just the word *body* is that it perpetuates a century-old misconception about Hatha Yoga that it applies *only* to the physical body. Despite his well-deserved reputation as a spiritual master, we can trace the seeds of this bad attitude about Hatha back to Swami Vivekananda. In his little book on the *Yoga-Sutra*, titled *Raja Yoga* and published in the late 1890s, the good, self-proclaimed swami wrote that Hatha Yoga "deals entirely with the physical body" and doesn't "lead to much spiritual growth."[4] Ouch. As we've already convincingly seen, despite being grounded in the physical body, Hatha Yoga clearly has its sights set on a spiritual goal. To more accurately represent the "pot" then, we should think of it as a *psycho*physical container, and *ghata* is better rendered as "body-mind."

Think about how a newly made pot, just off the potter's wheel and yet to be fired. If we immersed an unbaked or "raw" pot (*ama kumbha*) like this in water, it would quickly "perish" or "decay" (*sada*). Such is the condition of most people's bodies before they begin the practice of yoga that if they immediately immersed themselves in the higher practices of Hatha Yoga, such as *pranayama* and meditation, their bodies would be unprepared and fall apart like the unbaked pot. No matter how much we'd like to dive headfirst into the deep end of practice, our efforts would be fruitless, even perhaps injurious, unless our body-mind is first prepared or, as Gheranda famously remarks, "baked in the fire (*anala*) of yoga" (*Gheranda-Samhita* 1.8).

Probably the most widely known yoga system, that of Patanjali, has eight divisions, or "limbs" (*anga*). By contrast, Gheranda's union-method has seven, each of which leads to a specific result:

1. The "six acts" (*shat karma*) or purificatory rites lead to "cleanliness, purification, refinement" (*shodhana*). (Three of the acts are actually categories of practices rather than individual practices, so there are

about twenty acts altogether; see chapter 3.) These acts are, in a way, parallel in intent to Patanjali's *yamas* and *niyamas*. With the latter, you figuratively clean up your act by vowing to be, for example, non-violent, truthful, content, and self-aware; with the six acts, on the other hand, you literally do the housecleaning. Both disciplines then begin with a purification of their respective main arenas: with Patanjali, it's the consciousness (*chitta*); with Gheranda, the body.

2. Pose, or asana (see chapter 4), leads to "strength, fixedness, solidity" (*dridha*).

3. Seals (*mudras*) and their subset, bonds (*bandhas*; see chapter 6), lead to "firm, not wavering or tottering, steady; unfluctuating, durable, lasting, permanent; constant, steadfast, resolute, persevering" (*sthira*).

4. Sense withdrawal (*pratyahara*; literally "drawing back, retreat, withdrawal") leads to "self-possession, composure, calm" (*dhira*). Notice that in the *Gheranda-Samhita*, unlike the *Yoga-Sutra*, pratyahara precedes *pranayama*.

5. Conscious breathing (*pranayama*; see chapter 7) leads to "lightness, ease" (*aghava*).

6. Meditation (*dhyana*; see chapter 8) leads to "clear, distinct, manifest, direct, immediate, actual" perception (*pratyaksha*) of the self (*atman*).

7. *Samadhi* (see chapter 7) leads to purity (*nirlipta*; "unanointed, undefiled, unsullied") and "liberation, deliverance, beatitude" (*mukti*). Gheranda here uses the word *samadhina* instead of *samadhi*. Adhina means "to rest in or on," while the little *sama* has a host of denotations: "always the same, constant, unchanged, fair, impartial toward; having the right measure; equable, neutral, equally distant from extremes; just, upright, good, straight, honest; full, complete, whole, entire; peace."

LITTLE LAMP: *YAMA* AND *NIYAMA*

One question I'm often asked is, where are restraints (*yamas*) and injunctions (*niyamas*)? They're said to be so important as a practice foundation in Patanjali's system that many students wonder why none are mentioned here. Two answers come to mind: one is that Anonymous/ Gheranda didn't think them important, or two, he thought them so basic to the practice that he didn't feel it necessary to mention them. Svatmarama actually offers a number of somewhat scattered dos and don'ts that, taken together, add up to a Hatha *yama-niyama* list. Though we often have this picture of the yogi as a bag of bones whose main occupation is self-mortification, Svatmarama in fact warns us away from extreme austerities and emphasizes, for the time and place in which he was writing, moderation. He uses an interesting phrase in doing this: *niyama graha* ("to be seized by rigid restrictions or rules"), the latter word having the further implication of an "evil demon or spirit who seizes or exercises a bad influence on the body and mind of man." Both Svatmarama and Gheranda emphasize the importance of moderate diet (*mitahara*, or "measured eating"; see *Hatha-Yoga-Pradipika* 1.58–63, 2.14 and *Gheranda-Samhita* 5.16–32). Both suggest that eating should be a devotional act accompanied by, according to Gheranda, affection (*priya*) for the gods (*suras*). Practitioners should also avoid exertion and travel, not talk too much (*prajalpa*), and avoid socializing—especially with bad people and, of course, women. All this is no doubt designed to conserve as much energy as possible for practice.

On the positive side of the coin, Svatmarama praises enthusiasm (*utsaha*; "power, strength, resolution, effort, perseverance, energy, firmness, fortitude"); cheerfulness (*sahasa*; "accompanied with a laugh"); constancy (*dhairya*; "firmness, patience, calmness, gravity, fortitude); true knowledge (*jnana tattva*); courage (*nishcaya*; "inquiry, conviction, certainty, positiveness, resolution, resolve"); and solitude (*tyaga*). To this, Anonymous/Gheranda adds the absolute necessity of having conviction (*pratiti*; "confidence, faith, belief") in your own wisdom (*vidya*), in your guru, and in your self (*atman*) to awaken your mind (*manas*).

At this point, Gheranda's introduction is complete, and he launches into his practical teaching. Each division of the practice has its own chapter, the one on *pranayama* being the longest and the *pratyahara* chapter by far the shortest—and least interesting. The chapters are called *upadeshas* ("teachings, prescriptions"), which is plain enough, but the word also means "initiation, the communication of the initiatory mantra." In other words, each chapter isn't *just* a teaching; it's also a form of initiation into the mysteries of Hatha Yoga.

As we read along, remember that this initiation isn't to be taken lightly. In the old days, yoga could only be learned from a self-realized *guru,* and only after that *guru* accepted you into his circle through an initiatory ceremony. The ceremony usually proceeded through a half-dozen steps, which included an opening meditation on the guru by the candidate, a test of both the candidate's doctrinal knowledge and practical proficiency (e.g., in asana and pranayama), a symbolic funeral to mark the "death" of the student's old personality, a welcoming *abhisheka* or "anointing, consecrating" with water (like a baptism), and finally the transmission by the *guru.*

TURN OUT THE LIGHT: ABOUT THIS BOOK

Now that you have the background to Gheranda's teaching, we can begin the formal practice. What you'll find in chapter 2 is the energetic or imaginative foundation for all the subsequent practices in this book, and once learned, it can be applied to all of your yoga practice, no matter what kind. The work in this chapter isn't traditional, though I've tried to tie it tenuously to a traditional teaching about our subtle network of energetic "channels" (*nadi*). The information here is an amalgam from different modern sources and my own experience as a student for the last thirty years. These modern channels (or circuits, as I call them) are truly innate energetic patterns of the human body that apply at all times and in all places.

Chapters 3 and 5 through 8 address selected cleansing exercises (karma), Gheranda's thirty-two poses (asanas, with a few modifications), selected seals and bonds (mudras and *bandhas*), conscious breathing (*pranayama*), and meditation exercises. We'll run through all this material first, then I'll make some suggestions on how to put it into practice and how you can turn it into a personal practice in Appendix 1. Chapter 4 is more or less an introduction to the asana practice in chapter 5.

Speaking of asanas, I needed a way to illustrate the many poses mentioned in this book that aren't in the Original sequence without burdening the text with countless photographs. So I chose what you might consider a rather unorthodox way, especially if you're not an Iyengar or Iyengar-influenced student. I've used the plates in *Light on Yoga* to supplement the simple line drawings my artist rendered for the asana sequence in chapter 6. I assume that many students have around the house a copy of this famous book, with the silver cover and orange lettering. But if you don't, it's readily available online and in bookstores, or easily borrowed from a yoga friend or library.

2

CHANNELS
AND CIRCUITS:
MODERN *NADIS*

The mind (*manas*) becomes steady when the breath
(*marut*) moves in the middle (*madhya*).

—Hatha-Yoga-Pradipika 2.42

N A D I · the tubular stalk of any plant or
tubular organ (as a vein or an artery of the body);
any pipe or tube

MY COTTAGE in Berkeley, California—not quite as small as Gheranda's *matha*, but close—was built not long after the disastrous Bay Area earthquake in 1906. If I were to remove the inner walls of this charming but closet-space-challenged structure, I'd expose its wooden framework and a network of wires that zap electricity to each of my six rooms, along with pipes that carry water from the water heater in the back room to the kitchen and bathroom. The yogis call the outer covering of the body a "food sheath" (*anna maya kosha*)—the visible tip of the iceberg, so to speak—that encompasses four progressively more subtle sheaths of vital energy (*prana*), mind (*manas*), insight (*vijnana*), and bliss (*ananda*). They say that if we could remove this gross outer covering and open and peer through our mystic "third eye," we'd discern the delicate framework that holds us up and together. We are crisscrossed by tens of thousands of subtle "wires" and "pipes" (*nadis*)—Anonymous/Shiva compares them to "branches" (*shakha*) and "twigs" (*prashakha*)—that circulate vital energy (*prana*) to all of our nooks and crannies. These channels are connected through a line of "switching stations" called chakras ("wheels") that are arrayed vertically along the interior of the spine from its base at the sacrum to the crown (some say about a foot above the crown).

Only fourteen of the estimated seventy-two thousand *nadis* are principal; of these, just three are singled out for special notice in Hatha practice. At the top of this short list is the one located in the "middle" (*madhya*, cognate with our "middle"), exquisitely named the "most gracious channel" (*sushumna nadi*). It's the middle in two senses. First, in a general way, it's wrapped—like a wire's copper strands in rubber insulation—inside our physical spine, which in the secret or esoteric anatomy of Hatha is the middle of our body-mind. You may have heard the spine called the *meru danda* ("staff of Meru"), a phrase with a wealth of associations. Meru is the mythic mountain at the hub of the yogis' imaginative universe, around which the entire system revolves. Similarly, our spine is the hub of our miniature universe, an exact, though Lilliputian copy of its Brobdingnagian model. Second and more specifically, the *sushumna nadi* is in the middle of or between the two other main *nadis*: tawny (*pingala*; "reddish brown"), which represents the solar *ha* on the right side, and comfort (*ida*; "refreshing"), which represents the lunar *tha* on the left.

LITTLE LAMP: *DANDA*

The Sanskrit *danda* is typically translated as "staff" (as in Staff Pose, or *dandasana*). When referring to the spine then, it can symbolize the wandering ascetic's walking stick, which suggests the true seeker's dedication and humility, two essential elements of our practice. But *danda* can also mean "scepter," which suggests the power and authority that accrues to the practitioner of Hatha Yoga.

I'm not going to say much about subtle physiology or *kundalini*, even though they're of crucial importance in Hatha Yoga. These subjects, particularly the chakra system, have been greatly misunderstood and misused in the modern West. Considering the space limitations of this book, I fear I'd only be adding insult to injury if I tried to do the system justice. Besides at this point in our practice, when we're still dealing mostly with the physical body and its wildly rearing mind horses, tossing in simplified information about subtle anatomy isn't really of much use. Subtle teaching demands direct transmission from a living teacher; reading about it in a book without being able to ask or respond to questions can lead to all sorts of difficulties. However, if you're curious about the story behind *kundalini* and want to study it for yourself, have a look at *Layayoga: The Definitive Guide to the Chakras and Kundalini* by Shyam Sundar Goswami, the most extensive and traditionally correct book I've come across. If you want to challenge yourself to the maximum, because it's not an easy read, plow through the classic study by Sir John Woodroffe (writing as Arthur Avalon), *The Serpent Power: The Secrets of Tantric and Shaktic Yoga*.

IMAGINARY MOVEMENT

What I do intend to talk about is a system of what I call "modern *nadis*," inspired by a remarkable book published in the 1930s on human anatomy, posture, and movement titled *The Thinking Body* by Mabel Elsworth Todd. When I first read this book many years ago, I didn't understand that it outlined an open-ended body-work system that is now called Ideokinesis, or simply the Work. It's based on the premise that vivid images (ideo), if held in the mind's eye and focused on various parts or sections of the body (such as the shoulder blades or back pelvis) while lying completely still in what's called Constructive Rest Position, will promote postural and movement reeducation (kinesis). Luckily for me, one day I ran into an acquaintance who excitedly showed me some notes she'd taken while attending a local workshop taught by André Bernard, a student of one of Todd's students. Have you ever had a light bulb go off in your head? I was positively flabbergasted by these notes for three reasons. First, I'd completely missed the practical message of Todd's book. Second, those notes could just as easily have been taken in my regular yoga class, so perfectly did the information dovetail with what I was learning from my teacher at the time. Third, the central image of the

Work, an imaginative "line of energy" that constantly circulated—like Gheranda's waterwheel—up the front of the spine and down the back, was eerily similar to that of the awakened serpent power rising through the *sushumna nadi*.

LITTLE LAMP: ENERGY

I assume that most readers of this book accept the notion that, in yoga, we can talk about energy flowing through the body along a multitude of "energetic" channels. But I have to take into account the possibility that this volume will fall into the hands of a skeptic, specifically a scientific skeptic. If you belong to the former group, feel free to skip over this Lamp, but if you're the latter and you've made it this far, we need to talk. One of the biggest beefs scientific skeptics have with books like this one is the use—or in their estimation, misuse—of the word *energy*. I'm well aware that in scientific circles this word has a very precise meaning: a "scalar physical quantity that describes the amount of work that can be performed by a force," and so on. We yoga types may or may not know about scalar physical quantities, but we can feel, or at least imagine we feel, lines of what we can only define as energy coursing through our bodies. I understand this isn't energy in the scientific sense, and I can't define it as precisely as a scientifically trained mind would like; nevertheless, something is going on, even if it's an illusion. Let's just say then it's a very effective illusion. I'll ask you to have "yoga faith," as the nineteenth-century English poet Samuel Coleridge asked for "poetic faith," and for this practice, exercise what he called the "willing suspension of disbelief." Give these lines of energy a try, and you may find yourself coming over to the dark side.

My modern *nadis* are based in large part on the nine "essential lines of movement" developed by one of Todd's students, Lulu Sweigard, and described in her book *Human Movement Potential*. I also brought in material from the booklets of another of Todd's students, Barbara Clark, from my direct study with André on his yearly visit to Berkeley from his home in New York City and from several years of yoga classes. Without going into much detail, Sweigard's nine lines were the outcome of an experiment she conducted over several months on a group of female college students. First, she regularly guided the group through a series of Ideokinetic exercises that mapped specific images on their bodies — imagine the back of your pelvis opening up like an old-fashioned hand-held fan. Then, with a strange-looking contraption, she measured the effect on their posture. From the data she gathered about the women's physical changes, she extracted the ennead, at the heart of which is a line flowing up the front of the spine from the tailbone to the atlas (first cervical vertebra) and a companion line returning from that point back to the base of the spine.

With this as my starting point, I developed a network of imaginative, or energetic, channels that crisscross the body from head to foot. Most of these imaginative channels (except for that of the front spine and part of the head circuit) are on the surface of the body, so they can be traced with the hands and are, depending on the vividness of your imagination, more or less accessible. Taking Patanjali's pairs of opposites (*dvandvas;* see *Yoga-Sutra* 2.48) as my cue, I mated the channels up in pairs called circuits, some of which link up with others to create megacircuits. (Truthfully, not all of the circuits are exactly circular in their course; some look more like a pair of intersecting revolving wheels.) Unlike Patanjali, I prefer to call the mated channels "pairs of complements," and while classical yoga wants to transcend the opposites, I want to integrate the complements into my practice.

What purpose will these pairs serve in the upcoming practice? Generally the channels together serve as a coordinated network for routing imaginative energy through the body (unless there's a blockage in one of the channels, in which case the energy is prevented from flowing freely). Considered in toto, the channels support the two most basic urges of the human body-mind: (1) to descend into earth, or incarnate, and (2) to rise up into space, or transcend. Channels move in only one direction; most run vertically (in the standing position), but a few run horizontally or diagonally. Circuits (as the name suggests) are more or less circular, with no particular beginning or end, though often, for the sake of convenience, a starting place somewhere along the course of a circuit can be indicated. The head circuit, for example, will initiate from the occipital protuberance (see "Circuit 7: Head and Neck Circuit" later in this chapter). So most of the principal circuits of the body consist of two channels of energy flowing in opposite directions:

- The front spine flows up from the tailbone to the atlas at the bottom of the skull; the back spine flows down from the bottom of the skull back to the tailbone.
- The inner leg flows up from the inner ankle to the inner groin; the outer leg flows down from the outer hip to the outer ankle.
- The inner arm flows up (when the arms hang down) from the inner wrist to the inner armpit; the outer arm flows down from the outer armpit to the outer wrist. (Technically, the "front armpit" is the pectoralis major, the flap of muscle crossing the front shoulder from chest to arm. Similarly, in technical language, the "back armpit" is the latissimus dorsi, another muscle flap crossing the back shoulder.)

Each channel (or circuit) serves as what the yogis would call a support or prop (*adhara*), which Georg Feuerstein defines as "any of several places in the body on which the *yogin* focuses his attention not only to discipline the mind but also to harness the body's psychosomatic energy (*prana*)."[1] Traditionally a support was a specific spot in or on the body, but in contrast, my channels are *moving lines* of imaginary energy. As supports, they're more dynamic and more closely approximate the energetic nature of the body-mind.

My channels can be used in the following ways:

- As preparations (rehearsals) for movements at the start of a practice session
- To direct and/or harness energy during movement, and support both earth-embodiment and space-transcendence
- To create physical and psychological strength, alignment, and space
- As a focus for consciousness during relaxation at the end of practice

When I imagine these channels, I experience my body not as a fixed state, massive and opaque, but rather as a fluid process, "light" in both senses of the word's etymology (the Latin *levitas*, meaning "weightless," and the Greek *leukos*, meaning "illuminated"). Earlier I said I developed these lines, but that's not exactly what happened. It's more accurate to say that through a fortuitous concourse of events, I was fortunate enough to discover an energetic network inherent in the human body-mind. Like the scientists who predicted and then found certain elements based on early gaps in the periodic table, once I had a few of the lines mapped out, the others just fell into place. So the channels help me clarify, organize, and consolidate the manifold, often bickering voices of my body-mind. And because I'm assured by the yogis that I'm what we'd call today a hologram of the cosmos, these lines are universal, comprising principles that refer not only to my body-mind, but to the body-mind of the world I inhabit. Over time, the channels link up into an encompassing reality in which I am "put together"—the literal meaning of the word *samadhi*—with the self and its creation, so there is no longer any separation between the knower, the known, and the knowing. At least, that's what I like to imagine.

MODERN *NADIS*: A PRACTICE OVERVIEW

The exercises in this chapter are divided into eight circuits:

Circuit 1: Foot and Ankle Circuits
Circuit 2: Leg Circuit
Circuit 3: Hand Circuit
Circuit 4: Arm Circuit
Circuit 5: Pelvis Circuit
Circuit 6: Thorax Circuit
Circuit 7: Head and Neck Circuit
Circuit 8: Spine Circuit

Please work through each circuit in its proper order—no skipping allowed. As you will see, the sequence of exercises will take you "inward" from your periphery to your core, from your limbs to your torso to your spine. In this way, I hope you'll find the many parallels between different parts and limbs; the circuits of the legs and arms, for example, mirror each other. Although Sweigard's original lines of movement were applied imaginatively while lying in constructive rest, we'll work with the circuits a bit more dynamically, as much as is possible in full or modified yoga poses. Each circuit description includes a subcircuit application that gives you a few ideas on how to use it in the Original practice; however, I won't talk much about the circuits in the Original instructions themselves. I'll leave it to you to play with their possibilities.

LITTLE LAMP: ACTION AND MOVEMENT

Let me define two words before we begin. An *action* is an imaginary movement; for example, "lengthen your tailbone" is a call to action. A *movement,* on the other hand, is something physical; "stretch your arms over your head" is a call to move.

CIRCUIT 1: FOOT AND ANKLE CIRCUITS

The foot circuit combines channels running along the inner and outer edges of the foot. The inner foot channel runs from the mound of the big toe to the inner ankle; the outer foot channel runs from the outer heel along the outer edge of the foot and out through the little toe. The ankle circuit is a combination of two rotations: the inner ankle rotating outward (or laterally), and the outer ankle rotating inwardly (or medially).

Practice

From a standing position, exhale into Forward Bend (*uttanasana;* pose #18 in Iyengar's *Light on Yoga*). Bend your knees if you can't easily touch the floor with your knees fully straight. On the top of each foot, press your thumbs on the mounds of the big toes (but not the big toes themselves); imagine the big toes lengthening forward, away from the body of the foot. After 30 to 60 seconds, slide your thumbs away from the mounds along the inner edge of the feet to the inner ankles; repeat several times, keeping the big-toe mounds firm to the floor. Stroke *only* from the mounds of the big toes back to the ankles, never from the ankles to the big toes.

Once you have a feel for the inner foot channel, turn your attention to the outer foot. From the outer heels, stroke your fingers along the outer feet to the little toes. Once there, stroke away from the little toes, and just like the big toes, imagine them lengthening away from the foot into the room. Repeat several times, but as with the inner foot channel, stroke in *only* one direction, never back from the little toes to the heels.

Next, still in Forward Bend, hook your fingers under the same-side ankles, with your thumbs under the inner ankles and index fingers under the outer ankles. First, pull up on your ankles, as if trying to lift yourself off the floor. Be sure both inner ankles are lifted an equal distance from the floor. Then roll the inner anklebones out and the outer anklebones in, which will narrow the front of the ankle between the bones and widen the heel.

Benefit

The foot circuit enlivens the sole, making you more conscious of your contact with the floor while standing. This in turn helps you fine-tune the distribution of weight on and between your feet, so ideally your standing position will be more aligned and balanced, improving your posture and mobility. The ankle circuit strengthens your arches and, as the foundation of the front spine channel (see "Circuit 8: Spine Circuit" later in this chapter), creates a feeling of lightness through the energetic core of your body.

Application

These circuits are especially useful, of course, in the standing poses. There are only two standing poses in the Original sequence (Superior Pose and Tree Pose; see chapter 5), but there are at least two dozen in the modern repertoire.

LITTLE LAMP: SOLES AND SACRUM

The soles of the feet have energetic—or if you prefer, imaginary—connections with the sacrum (just as the hands do with the shoulder blades). The sacrum, you may already know, is the bone, shaped like an inverted triangle, that serves as both the back of the pelvis and base of the spine.

For this exercise, imagine dividing your sacrum into left and right halves, drawing a line from the midpoint at the top of the bone (technically and somewhat confusingly called its base) straight down through the tailbone. The right sole is energetically in sympathy with the right side of the bone, and the left sole with the left side. Still standing in Forward Bend, bring your hands to your sacrum. As you spread your right sole on the floor and trigger the foot circuit, use your right hand to slide the right side of the sacrum away from the midline. (You needn't do anything more than this right now; we'll complete the action of widening later.) Now do the same with your left sole and left-side sacrum, then try both soles and both sides of the sacrum simultaneously. This should further sensitize your soles and, at the same time, help release your torso into a deeper forward bend.

CIRCUIT 2: LEG CIRCUIT

The leg circuit combines channels running along the inner and outer legs. The inner leg channel runs from the inner ankle to the inner groin (where the inner thigh joins the base of the pelvis, or perineum); the outer leg channel runs down from the outer hip along the outer leg to the heel.

Practice

In standing Forward Bend, slowly stroke up along your inner legs from the ankles all the way to the perineum. Repeat several times, being sure to stroke slowly and in only one direction. Then bring your hands to your outer hips; from there, slowly stroke down your outer legs several times, stopping at the outer ankles each time.

Now let's join the foot, ankle, and leg circuits. Bring your thumbs back to the mounds of the big toes. Press down, then slowly stroke along the inner feet to the inner ankles, loop your thumbs around the inner ankles, and slide them up the inner legs to the perineum. From here bring your hands to the outer hip and stroke down along the outside of your legs to the outer ankles, loop under the anklebones and continue along the outer feet. Finish by imagining lengthening out through the little toes. Repeat several times.

Benefit

The inner leg channel is an energetic continuation of the inner ankle, a line of energy that feeds into the energetic front spine (see "Circuit 8: Spine Circuit" later in this chapter) and continues out through the crown to a point above the head. This upward-flowing energy through the core of your entire body creates a centered feeling of lightness and ease. The outer leg channel helps return all the high-flying energy back to the floor—or if you prefer, the earth.

Application

As with the foot circuit, the leg circuit is especially useful in standing poses. But the inner leg channel is applicable across the board in just about every other pose. All the sitting poses, for example, always draw energetically along the inner thigh from the knee to the groin. This action should initiate the forward bend in, say, Intense-Stretch-of-the-West Pose (*pashchima uttanasana*; see chapter 5).

BLOCK AND THIGHS

Preparation

Stand in Mountain Pose. Turn your thighs outward (laterally), that is, rotate from the inner thigh to the outer. Your feet may want to turn outward a bit, Charlie Chaplin–style, but prevent them for doing so. Now turn your thighs inward (medially), that is, rotate from the outer thigh to the inner. Your feet may now want to go pigeon-toed, but keep them steady on the floor. Repeat a few times, turning out, then in.

Practice

You can practice this exercise with a block squeezed between your thighs. Use the narrowest width of the block, and keep the top of it a few inches below your perineum. In the anatomical world, when you squeeze a block like this between your thighs, you're using your inner thigh muscles (adductors), but in the yoga world, we pretend we're using the *outer* thigh muscles (abductors). I want to emphasize that this is all imaginary; we pretend so we can create an effect in the feet. Be careful as you squeeze the block, that you don't harden the outer hips. Turn the thighs inward slightly, that is, roll the block toward whatever's behind you.

From Mountain, exhale and tip your torso into a forward bend. Start by pressing your hands against your outer thighs to give yourself a feel for the inward firming of the outer thighs. In the best of all possible worlds, this action will accentuate the firmness of the mounds of your big toes on the floor. From this contact, draw back to the inner ankles and lift up through the inner ankles.

CIRCUIT 3: HAND CIRCUIT

The hand channels mirror the foot channels, the mound of the index finger being analogous to the mound of the big toe and the little finger being analogous to the little toe.

Preparation

Look at your right palm. With the tip of your left index finger, press on the mound of the right index finger. Hold the press steady for 15 to 20 seconds. Now shift your attention to the base of the palm. To the right is the mound of the thumb; to the left, the mound of the little finger. Spread your fingers broadly, and in between these two mounds is a slight indentation on the base of your palm that I call the "hollow." Rub your left index finger back and forth along this hollow several times, imagining that by doing so you're deepening it between the mounds to either side, like a valley between two hills. Finally, imagine that the circumference of your palm (excluding the fingers) is shaped like a circle, and with the tip of your left index finger, press firmly in its exact center. Hold the pressure steady for 15 to 20 seconds. Repeat the entire exercise with the hands reversed.

Practice

From standing Forward Bend, kneel down on your mat and sit back on your heels for a moment. Now press your left palm to the floor with the fingers pointing forward away from your torso. Just as you did with the mound of your big toe, press the mound of your index finger firmly to the floor. You can use the fingers of your right hand to press down on the index finger knuckle to accentuate the feeling of pressure. As you ground the mound of your index finger, actively lift the hollow between the mounds of the thumb and little fingers and the center of the circular-shaped palm. This should ideally shift more weight onto the index finger mound and lighten the pressure on your wrist. Finally, as you did with the outer edge of your foot and little toe, stroke along the outer edge of your hand and imagine your little finger lengthening out along the floor. Continue for a minute or so, then repeat with the hands reversed.

Benefit

Like the foot circuit, the hand circuit enlivens the hands and, when bearing weight, relieves pressure on the wrists. Combined with the arm circuit, it creates strength and stability.

Application

Use these exercises in palms-on-the-floor poses, like Rooster Pose and Peacock Pose, in the Original sequence (see chapter 5) to help take weight off the wrists. When all your weight is borne on the hands as in these poses, the hand circuit will also help to stabilize the pose.

PALMS AND SHOULDER BLADES

Just as the soles of the feet are energetically connected to the sacrum, the palms are connected to the shoulder blades. There's really no good way to make a tactile-aided connection on your own, as you did with the soles and your hands on the sacrum. If you have a yoga partner, you can try this experiment. Stand facing a blank wall. Press and spread your palms on the wall, elbows straight, hands at shoulder height and equidistant from the floor, index fingers parallel to each other or slightly turned out. Have your partner press and spread her hands on your shoulder blades. First you both focus on the right shoulder blade — you while spreading your palm on the wall, your partner while spreading her hand on your shoulder blade. Take a minute or so to see if you can make the connection, then shift your attention to the left palm and shoulder blade for a minute. When you feel ready, try both shoulder blades together, first with your partner's hands in place, then solo.

Remember that your outer arms are analogous to your outer legs. When you spread your shoulder blades as if they were palms, you may feel them widening across your back, as though they were moving away from the spine and wrapping around the side of your torso. As you feel this, re-create what you felt in your outer thighs during the block-squeezing exercise in your outer arms. Firm them inward against the widening of the shoulder blades.

CIRCUIT 4: ARM CIRCUIT

The arm channels mirror the leg channels, which can be summarized as "up the inner, down the outer."

Practice

Still in the kneeling position, press your left palm to the floor as instructed for the hand circuit, with your arm fully extended (elbow straight) and more or less perpendicular to the floor. With the fingers of your right hand, slowly stroke up your inner left arm from the wrist to the inner armpit, then — just as you did with the leg circuit — stroke down your outer arm from the outer armpit to the outer wrist. Repeat several times, then repeat with the arms reversed.

Now let's join the hand and arm circuits. Still kneeling — or moving into Downward-Facing Dog Pose (*adho mukha shvanasana; Light on Yoga* #33) even though it's not part of the Original sequence — once again press your left palm to the floor as instructed for the hand circuit. From the mound of the index finger, energetically draw back to the inner wrist, then from the inner wrist draw up along the inner arm to the inner armpit. Shift your awareness across to the outer armpit, and from there, lengthen down the outer arm to the outer wrist. At the same time, firm the outer arm inward as you did in the preceding Little Lamp. If you like, you can now press against your left biceps with your right hand. Finally, lengthen along the outer edge of the hand, as you did with the foot.

Benefit

This exercise strengthens the arms in the palms-on-the-floor poses (again like Rooster Pose and Peacock Pose in the Original sequence).

Preparation: Arm Rotation

Stretch your right arm straight out in front of your torso. Turn it outward (laterally) so the palm faces up, then inward (medially) so the palm faces down. Repeat a few times, turning out, then in.

Practice

Press your left hand to the floor as instructed for the arm circuit. Now rotate the upper arm outward. As you do this, the weight on your palm will shift to the little-finger side. Once you've established this rotation, hold it and roll the weight on your palm across the bases of the fingers to the mound of the index finger. Feel how, as the upper arm rolls outward, the forearm rotates in the opposite direction (inward) to bring the index mound firmly to the floor.

Repeat this exercise with your right hand, then lift into Downward-Facing Dog Pose (as in Circuit 4) to work both arms simultaneously.

CIRCUIT 5: PELVIS CIRCUIT

The pelvis circuit is the model for the ankle circuit and anchors the circuit of the rest of the torso. We can summarize it as follows: wide across the back, narrow across the front. Let's define a few landmarks to make sure the following directions are clear.

Preparation

You've already found the midline of your sacrum in your mind's eye. Now with a thumb, start somewhere on the middle of your lower back and stroke a line down across the sacrum to your tailbone, ideally dividing the sacrum into right and left halves. Now press your fingertips a few inches to either side of your navel and find a pair of little bony knobs. These are the hip points.

Practice

Lie on your back, preferably on a sticky mat, and be sure you have a yoga block handy. On an exhalation, bend your knees and draw your thighs to your belly, then wrap your arms around your shins or the back of your thighs, whichever is easier. Now rock gently and slowly from side to side. As you do, imagine the back of your pelvis widening away from its midline — right side to the right, left side to the left. Continue for a minute or two, then slowly come to a stop and lightly touch your feet to the floor, big toes turned slightly in. Next bring your hands to your hip points and firmly press them toward each other, so that as the back of your pelvis continues to widen, the front pelvis narrows. Hold this for a minute or two.

Now press your feet into the floor and lift your pelvis off the floor. Slide the block at its lowest height underneath your sacrum, with its long axis parallel to your spine. Lay your pelvis down on the block, making sure the tailbone is supported. Again, rock slowly from side to side, imagining as you do that the block is gently pressing your sacrum deeper into the back of your pelvis. Continue for a minute or two, then stop in what you experience to be the midway point between the two extremes of rocking. Rest here for another minute or two. With each exhalation, imagine the block pressing the sacrum deeper into the pelvis without narrowing the back pelvis.

Now let's integrate the circuits of the feet, legs, and pelvis. Return to a standing Forward Bend, feet hip-width apart. Bring your hands to the back of your pelvis on the sacrum and slowly stroke each hand away from the sacrum toward the same-side hip, widening the buttock muscles to the sides. Stop at the outer hips for 30 seconds or so. With your hands in loose fists, gently "fluff" your outer hips as you would a pair of down-filled pillows. Then slide your hands across to the front of your pelvis and press the hip points toward each other.

Once the front of your pelvis is narrowed, return your hands to the outer hips; from here, stroke slowly down the outer legs, pressing firmly inward as you go, as if to press the outer legs together. When you reach the ankles, grip them as you did in Circuit 1 and pull up, trying to lift yourself off the floor (which would happen if the mounds of your big toes weren't glued to the floor with yoga glue). Now slowly stroke up the inner legs to the inner groins and perineum. Here bring your hands to the floor just in front of your feet (bend your knees if needed), and supporting your weight on your hands, lift your heels about an inch off the floor. As you do, you'll feel added pressure on the mounds of the big toes, which will help you get an even better feel for pressing them to the floor.

With your heels still elevated, imagine lifting from the inner ankles along the inner legs to the inner groins and, once there, drawing the inner groins up into and through the pelvis toward the sacrum. When the energetic lift reaches this bone, spread it across the back of the pelvis; as you feed it down the outer legs toward the heels, and without losing the height of the inner groins, slowly press your heels back to the floor. Repeat this sequence a few more times using your hands. Then press your hands back to the floor and repeat again using just your imagination to stroke along the circuits, up the inner legs from the ankles to the inner groin, down the outer legs from the hips to the outer heels.

Benefit

The widening of the back pelvis helps to release your back. The narrowing of the front pelvis firms your abdomen and helps lengthen your spine.

Application

Widening the back pelvis protects your back during backbends, preventing the lower (lumbar) back from overarching.

Circuit 6: Thorax Circuit

The thorax, or rib case, circuit follows the lead of the pelvis circuit and is summed up as follows: wide across the back, narrow across the front, with the exception of the collarbones.

Practice

Lie on your back and repeat the bent-knee exercise that began Circuit 5. Rock slowly from side to side and feel your entire back torso widening away from your spine, the midline of the back. After a minute or two, set your feet on the floor and keep your knees bent.

Bring your hands onto your side ribs and gently stroke across the side and front ribs to the sternum (breastbone). Repeat several times. Now imagine the two sides of the back torso widening away from the spine and, at the same time, the front ribs narrowing in toward the sternum.

This narrowing of the front ribs would cause the chest to sink were it not for the collarbones, which provide a countermovement to the ribs. So as the front ribs continue to narrow from the sides of the torso toward the sternum, lay your fingertips on your collarbones — right hand on right collarbone, left hand on left — so the little fingers are near the sternum and the index fingers near the outer tips of the bones. Firmly spread the bones away from the sternum toward the tips of the shoulders, and at the same time, firmly push them up toward the tops of the shoulders. Imagine a space opening between your collarbones and the top ribs, which pass directly underneath them. As you lift your collarbones toward the top of your shoulders, gently press your feet against the floor, as if trying to push yourself in the direction of your head (but don't physically move). As you do this, you'll ideally feel your shoulder blades pressed down the back torso toward the tailbone. Imagine feeding the lifting collarbones into the descending shoulder blades, which continue in your mind down your back toward the tailbone. Remember that the spread of the collarbones shouldn't come at the expense of the width of the shoulder blades; in other words, the width you feel across your upper chest should match the width you feel across your upper back.

Finally, imagine two wheels attached to your shoulder, parallel to the spine, so their axle runs across your shoulders from side to side. Watch as these wheels turn up the front of your torso and down the back, assisting the lift of the collarbones and descent of the shoulder blades.

Benefit

This action helps to lift your front torso and lengthen your front spine.

LITTLE LAMP: THE STERNUM

Have you ever been asked to lift your chest, your sternum, or your heart during a yoga class? When following this instruction, it's important to distinguish between the top of the sternum and the bottom. The top of the bone is the manubrium (from the Latin for "handle"), the bottom is the xiphoid (from the Greek for "sword"), and the body of the bone is the gladiolus (from the Latin *gladius*, or "sword"). Taking these names as our cue, we can visualize the sternum as a knife, its handle at the base of the throat, its sharp tip pointing downward toward the navel. Typically, when given the instruction to lift the sternum, a student will lift the *bottom* of the bone, pushing the xiphoid forward and up, overarching the lower back, squeezing the shoulder blades together, and actually *dropping* the upper chest slightly. What's needed instead is to visualize the "knife" on your chest and pull its "handle" straight up while holding its tip in toward the torso and lengthening it down toward the navel. While the overall movement of the chest is far less obvious, the actual lift is far more effective and healthier. You can ground this lift by simultaneously lengthening your tailbone toward the floor (in the standing position).

CIRCUIT 7: HEAD AND NECK CIRCUIT

The head circuit turns in the opposite direction of the spine circuit (see the next section, "Circuit 8: Spine Circuit"), that is, up the back and down the front. Let's define a few landmarks to make sure the following directions are clear.

Preparation

First touch a fingertip to the hollow at the top of your sternum and the bottom of the front of your throat. This is called the jugular notch in Western anatomy and the "well of the throat" (*kantha kupe*) by the yogis. Patanjali says that by meditating on this depression (*Yoga-Sutra* 3.30), you'll overcome all hunger and thirst. Next slip your fingertip up to the crease where the underside of your chin joins the front of your throat. This is what I call the crook of the throat. Slide your fingertip back and forth along this crease a few times. The hyoid bone, which supports the root of the tongue, is just underneath.

Now touch the little bumps on the sides of your nose. These are the alae (singular *ala,* Latin for "wing"), or wings of the nose. Press the tip of your tongue to the roof of your mouth, or the hard palate. Can you reach it back far enough to touch the soft palate at the back of your throat?

Find the bony base of the back of your skull, just above the soft nape. There's a small natural bump back there called the occipital protuberance (because it's on the occiput bone), also known as the inion (Greek for "back of the neck"). Finally, slide your hand around on the top of your head. This is the crown; directly beneath it, inside your head, is the cranial vault.

While a circuit can begin anywhere along its course, we'll begin the head circuit at the inion.

Practice

Stay on your back, knees bent, feet on the floor. Lift your head slightly and poke around with the fingers of both hands until you can feel the inion; maintaining contact with your fingertips, lay your head back down on the floor. Now slide your fingertips up the back of your head to the crown and from there down across your forehead, dragging the forehead skin from the hairline to the bridge of your nose, across your inner eyes, across the wings of your nose, across the outer corners of your mouth, over your chin, and down to the crook of your throat. With your index fingertips touching this crease on either side of the larynx, gently press in and up (that is, diagonally); imagine taking a line of energy through your head and back to the starting point at the base of your skull. Repeat several times, each time saying the head circuit mantra to yourself: "up the back, down the front."

To accentuate the lift of the back skull, bring your fingertips to the back of your neck, just below the inion. As you continue to imagine lifting the back of your head, stroke down on the back of your neck. Imagine a space opening like an eye between the back skull and the back neck.

Repeat several times, imagining that the downward flow of the back neck continues along the back torso and finally out through the tailbone.

Benefit

The traditional books talk about the mystical "third eye" located at the bridge of the nose between the eyebrows. However, I like to imagine this eye at the base of my skull, opening wide in wonder and amazement at the beauty of the world as I spread the space between the inion and the nape. The benefits of this opening are legion. First, of course, it releases tension at the back of the neck and helps align a "forward head" over the spine where it belongs. What's a forward head? Next time you're in yoga class, or even out and about in the nonyoga world, look at a few people standing near you from the side. Draw an imaginary line from their ear canal through the center of their shoulder, center of their hip, and center of their ankle. Is that line more or less perpendicular to the floor or ground? Ideally, it should be. What you'll typically find is that the ear canal, and thus the head, is slightly *ahead* of where it should be relative to the rest of the body. That's a forward head, which is hanging off the spine instead of balancing on it, causing the back neck muscles to contract to hold its weight up. This results in a host of physical problems, most prominently nagging headaches. Opening the so-called third eye helps bring the head back over the spine to relieve neck tension.

But there are more positive consequences. The opening also helps to soften the soft palate and the back of the throat and to draw the crook of the throat diagonally in and up toward the atlas. This in turn softens the tongue (which is rooted in the hyoid) and magnetically pulls the manubrium upward. Seen from the side, there is a figure-eight circuit in the head and upper torso: from the inion to the crown and down across the face to the crook of the throat; from here, the circuit splits, with half going back through the head to the inion and half passing down through the throat to the tops of the shoulder blades. There the energy descends to the blades' lower tips and then ascends diagonally through the torso to the manubrium, where it reinforces from below the lift created from above by the opening of the third eye. At the manubrium, the energy continues up to the crook of the throat and so back to the inion.

Application

The head circuit applies across the board to all the poses. It's an essential preparation for Shoulderstand (see chapter 5) and the Net-Bearing Bond (see chapter 6).

LITTLE LAMP: EAR CIRCUIT

The small ear circuit mirrors the larger head circuit and can help accentuate the latter's action. Before we begin, let's define two ear terms to help get ourselves situated. The body of the ear is called the pinna (from the Latin for "feather") or auricle (from the Latin *auricula*, or "ear"), the little bump in from of the ear canal is the tragus (from the Greek *tragos*, or "goat"). Lightly touch your right index fingertip to the back of the same-side pinna just above the lobe. Slowly trace the outline of the pinna, sliding up to the top and then down past the tragus, looping around the lobe and back to the starting point. Repeat several times on the right ear, then make the circuit the same number of times on the left. Finally, imagine two little pinwheels, one on either side of your head, spinning up the back and down the front; in other words, looked at from the side, the right wheel rotates clockwise and the left one counterclockwise. These little wheels will complement and support the movement of the head circuit.

LITTLE LAMP: EYE CIRCUIT

Yes, even the eye has a circuit. Close your eyes and touch the tip of your right index finger *gently* to the inner corner of your right eye (just beside the nose). Stroke lightly across the lower edg of the socket to the outer corner, then back across the upper edge, just below the eyebrow, and back to the starting point. Repeat several times on the right, then the same number of times on the left eye. Now stroke in this way around both eyes simultaneously. Finish by visualizing a pair of rotating wheels around the rims of your eyes; looking from "inside" your head, the left wheel rotates clockwise and the right wheel counterclockwise.

CIRCUIT 8: SPINE CIRCUIT

Just as Mount Meru is the hub of the yogis' mythic universe, so is the spine circuit the hub of our "wheel" of modern *nadis*. Like most of the other circuits, the spine circuit consists of a pair of channels flowing in opposite directions along the front and back spines. You can run a fingertip along the back spine channel, which descends along the tips of the vertebrae from the base of the skull to the tailbone. There are two front spines, one physical and the other "metaphysical" or imaginary, neither of which you can physically touch. The physical front spine follows the line of the vertebrae, which are naturally buried deep in the torso. The metaphysical front spine is a line of imaginary energy ascending from the middle of the perineum at the base of the pelvis to the center of the crown. This line is actually a continuation of the inner thigh channels, which draw energy from the earth. When the line reaches the crown, we'll follow Hatha tradition and extend up through the head to a point about a foot above called the "end of twelve" (*dvadasha anta*), because it's measured by twelve finger widths.

Because it can be difficult to trace the front spine channel at first, we'll shift our focus to the front torso, where it's easy enough to run a fingertip up from the pubis to the top of the sternum. This will give you a feel for the action of the front spine channel. As you become more in tune with the front torso, you can eventually transfer the feeling to the imaginary line at the torso's core.

Practice

Lie on your back with your knees bent, feet on the floor, arms out to the sides, palms up (make sure you're on your sticky mat), and eyes closed. Lightly press your feet against the floor, as if trying to slide yourself in the direction of your head, but don't physically move. The pressure of your feet will scrub your back torso downward from the shoulders to the tailbone. This will give you a general feel for the descent of the back spine channel. Be careful here: the foot pressure will also pull the back of your head down, jutting your chin toward the ceiling. Be sure to keep your chin slightly tucked and the back of your neck long.

As you continue to press your feet against the floor and scrub your back downward, lightly trace a fingertip upward along your front torso from the pubis to the top of the sternum. Repeat several times. This is the basic action of the front spine channel.

If you feel confident and want to take it further, cross your arms over your torso, holding each shoulder with the opposite hand. Now rock gently from side to side, imagining your torso is shaped like a cylinder (it's not, but pretend). When you have a feel for that shape, stop rocking. In your mind, draw a line through the bottom of the cylinder (perineum) to the top (midshoulders) to represent the front spine. As you continue to press your feet and scrub your back downward, watch the imaginary front spine ascend through the cylinder, feed over the shoulders and into the back spine channel; when it reaches the tailbone, it reverses course and feeds into the front spine. And so around and around it goes — up the front, down the back.

Now roll to your side and stand up. Place your feet a few inches apart, parallel to each other, the ball of each foot spread wide. Let your arms hang comfortably alongside your torso. Press the mounds of your big toes firmly to the floor, energetically draw back from there along the inner feet to the inner ankles, then loop up along the inner legs to the groins. From here, continue the energetic line up into your torso, following either the front torso or the imaginary front spine. At your shoulders, you can do one of two things. If you're not quite ready to go full tilt with this exercise, feed the energy over the shoulders and into the back spine channel, through the tailbone, and into the earth all the way down to its core.

But if you feel ready to work a bit more subtly, when the energy reaches your shoulders, imagine that it divides. Half the stream flows into the back channel as already described, but the other half continues upward through your head. When it reaches the crown, it passes out through an opening the yogis call the "Brahma hole" (*brahma randhra*) and continues to the aforementioned terminus at the end of twelve. This image gives your body and head a feeling of being lifted from below, "pushed up" from the earth rather than "pulled up" from the sky.

Whichever circuit version you work with, stay in the standing pose for a few minutes, tracing the circuits in your imagination.

Benefit

The spine circuit creates a feeling of lightness and integration through-out your body.

Application

The spine circuit is the Meru of all the poses and breathing exercises. But more than that, it's also at the hub of our daily universe. Whatever you do in your practice or daily life, remember the mantra "up the front, down the back."

TURN OUT THE LIGHT

As I mentioned in the first chapter, these modern *nadis* supply the en-ergetic foundation, not only for the specific practice in this book, but for your entire yoga practice. Once you've worked with them for a while, you'll find yourself naturally observing their flow around and through your body as you go about your daily business; it's a kind of walking, running, sitting, standing, and even lying-down meditation. You'll find yourself making continuous small adjustments to your body based on these circuits that will keep you in tip-top physical alignment.

3

THE SIX ACTS
(*SHAT KARMA*)

The "six acts" should be kept hidden (*gopya*). They
purify the body and bestow "strange and wonderful"
(*vichitra*) qualities. As a result they are revered (*puja*)
by the most eminent (*pungava*) yogis.

—A loose translation of *Gheranda-Samhita 2.23*

THE PURIFICATORY PRACTICES

SHASH • six

KARMA • act, action, performance; any religious act or rite

The first two limbs of Patanjali's eight-limb system are the well-known "restraints" (*yama*) and "observances" (*niyama*). Proponents of this system believe that until you figuratively clean up your act—make nonviolence (*ahimsa*), truthfulness (*satya*), contentment (*santosha*), and all the rest the foundation of your life—it isn't possible to practice Patanjali Yoga successfully. For Gheranda's form of yoga of the Pot (and Svatmarama's *pranayama*) a preliminary housecleaning is recommended too, though instead of a set of behavioral injunctions, the "six acts" (*shat karma*) are hygienic practices, some as simple as massaging your gums and cleaning your ears, others as complicated as . . . well, we'll come to that soon. Let me first explain a couple of things about the number six and the translation of the Sanskrit word *karma* as "act," both of which are somewhat misleading.

LITTLE LAMP: KARMA

Like many words in yoga's Sanskrit lexicon, *karma* can't easily be rendered into English with just one word. It does indeed mean "act" or "performance," which tells us in this context that something concrete is being done. But *karma* also suggests that even the simplest act, if performed with devotion, has ritual or sacrificial dimension that transforms us not only physically but psychologically and spiritually. The paradox here is that what we're ultimately "sacrificing" are just those qualities of ourselves that stand in the way of our own self-realization. Gheranda tells us the end result of the six acts is *shodhana,* which means both "cleaning, purifying" and "correcting, improving, refining."

Gheranda positions the acts as the first stage of his seven-stage system and covers them in about fifty verses. In contrast, Svatmarama's six acts are six and only six; for him, *dhauti, basti,* Neti, Trataka, Nauli, and *kapala bhati* are all individual practices, and they're positioned between asana and *pranayama* in the *Hatha-Yoga-Pradipika.* Apparently though, not all the teachers of Svatmarama's time were convinced of the usefulness of the acts, or at least their usefulness for all practitioners. He cites two camps that held opposing views: one felt that the acts were necessary only for those practitioners with too much fat (*meda*) or mucus (*shlesma*); another believed that *pranayama* alone was sufficient to purify the body-mind, so the acts were superfluous.

Traditional Benefit

I'll go into more detail later about the benefits of these practices, but in general, they're supposed to purify and beautify the body, stoke the digestive "fire," balance the body's humors, "destroy" a variety of diseases (such as coughing, asthma, an enlarged spleen or abdominal tumor, leprosy) and forestall old age and death. Now before you rush off to start Gheranda's Six Acts Program for a Healthy, Happy, and Eternal You, I want to emphasize that not all of these practices are suitable for everyone, and several should only be attempted under the supervision of an experienced teacher.

LITTLE LAMP: SIX (*SHASH*)

The word *six* needs to be clarified too, but not as a translation of *shash*, which only means "six." Of the six names for the acts, only three refer to single exercises, the other three are general headings for two or more exercises. So Cleaning (*dhauti*), the first act listed, is a general heading for four subheadings, among which are distributed twelve practices. Bladder or Lower Belly (*basti*, also spelled *vasti*), the second act, is the heading for two practices, and Skull Brightening (*kapala bhati*) heads up three practices. The three single acts are those whose Sanskrit names have no adequate English rendering, and consequently they're usually left untranslated: Neti, which cleans the nasal sinuses; Nauli, which pumps the abdomen; and Trataka, which cleans the eyes. Add all these up (12 + 2 + 3 + 3), and we have a grand total of twenty practices that make up the six acts. All clear? (By the way, you might be wondering why or how the Sanskrit "six," which is *shash* by itself, turns into *shat* in combination with the word *karma*. It's a very long story, but essentially the last letter of the word, the retroflex *s* as it's called in Sanskrit, which is transliterated into the Roman alphabet as *sh*, is magically transformed into a *t* when it butts up against the *k* of *karma*.)

THE SIX ACTS: PRACTICE OVERVIEW

In the practice — sections 1 through 6 that follow — I've arranged the acts according to their applicable body part, that is, skull, eyes, nose, ears, mouth (teeth, tongue, throat), and belly. Section 7 briefly describes the remaining acts, which apply to the abdominal area and should only be performed under the supervision of a living teacher.

Section 1: Skull
    Skull Cleaning (*kapala dhauti*; *Gheranda-Samhita* 1.33–34)
    Skull Brightening (*kapala bhati*; *Hatha-Yoga-Pradipika* 2.35;
        Gheranda-Samhita 1.54–59)
Section 2: Eyes
    Trataka (*Hatha-Yoga-Pradipika* 2.31–32; *Gheranda-Samhita* 1.52)
Section 3: Nose and Sinuses
    Water Neti (*jala neti*)

Section 4: Ears
    Ear Cleaning (*karna dhauti; Gheranda-Samhita* 1.32)
Section 5: Teeth, Tongue, and Throat
    Cleaning the Root of the Teeth (*danta mula dhauti; Gheranda-Samhita* 1.26–27)
    Tongue Cleaning (*jihva dhauti; Gheranda-Samhita* 1.28–31)
    Cleaning with a Stick (*danda dhauti; Gheranda-Samhita* 1.36–37)
    Cleaning by Vomiting (*vamana dhauti; Gheranda-Samhita* 1.38)
Section 6: Belly
    Fire-Moving Cleaning (*vahni sara dhauti; Gheranda-Samhita* 1.19–20)
Section 7: Miscellaneous Acts (for Information Only)
    Air-Moving Cleaning (*vata sara dhauti; Gheranda-Samhita* 1.15–16)
    Water-Moving Cleaning (*vari sara dhauti; Gheranda-Samhita* 1.17–18)
    Expelled Cleaning (*bahish krita dhauti; Gheranda-Samhita* 1.21–24)
    Cleaning with a Cloth (*vaso dhauti; Hatha-Yoga-Pradipika* 2.24–25; *Gheranda-Samhita* 1.39–40)
    Root Purifying (*mula shodhana; Gheranda-Samhita* 1.41–43)
    Wet Bladder (*jala vasti; Hatha-Yoga-Pradipika* 2.27–28; *Gheranda-Samhita* 1.45–46)
    Dry Bladder (*shushka vasti; Gheranda-Samhita* 1.47–48)
    Nauli (*Hatha-Yoga-Pradipika* 2.33–34; *Gheranda-Samhita* 1.51)

SECTION 1: SKULL

SKULL CLEANING (KAPALA DHAUTI)

KAPALA · skull (also cognate with "capital, decapitate, captain")
DHAUTA · washed, cleaned, purified

Practice

Use your right thumb to rub the *bhala randhra,* about which my sources once again part interpretive ways. Two of them translate the Sanskrit as the aperture (*randhra*) at the roof of the mouth (*bhala*). This means you use your right thumb to massage the hollow in the roof of the palate.

The problem with this is that my dictionary and two other sources translate *bhala* as "forehead." They say you're to rub the slight depression or channel in your forehead at the root or bridge of the nose. We'll go with the latter translation.

Gheranda doesn't give any details about this rubbing—how long, how hard, whether it should be up and down, back and forth, or circular. Since the channel we're talking about is vertical (that is, perpendicular to the line across the eyebrows), let's assume that we should rub it up and down with moderate pressure for a few minutes.

Gheranda advises that Skull Cleaning should be done daily after waking up, after eating, and at day's end. Shri Yogendra, a contemporary teacher, recommends rubbing for about a minute each time.

Traditional Benefit

This practice purifies the subtle energy channels (*nadis*) and confers "divine sight" (*divya drishti*). It also serves as a preliminary to *shambhavi mudra* (see chapter 8).

LITTLE LAMP: GLABELLA THE HAIRLESS

The area at the bridge of the nose in Western anatomy is called the glabella, literally "hairless" (the word is related to *glabrous,* which means "bald," so our palms and soles are said to be thus). The skin here is attached directly to the frontalis muscle underneath, a muscle that helps open the eyes, raise the eyebrows, and furrow our worry lines. Biofeedback practitioners use the frontalis to monitor muscular tension, and some studies seem to indicate that purposive relaxation of the frontalis helps reduce headaches and anxiety for certain people.

SKULL BRIGHTENING (KAPALA BHATI)

BHATI · light, splendor; perception, knowledge

This exercise is also called Brow Brightener (*bhala bhati*), Head Brightener (*mastaka bhati*), and Skull Purifier (*kapala shodhana*). According to Gheranda, there are three kinds of *kapala bhati*. In the Air Process (*vata krama;* 1.55–56), breathing is done through alternate nostrils; in other words, inhale through the left nostril and exhale through the right, then reverse. Do this quickly (*vega*) and don't hold the breath. Svatmarama has a slightly different take on this practice. He says to empty (*recha*) and fill (*pura*) the lungs "hurriedly" (*sambrahma*), like a blacksmith's bellows, but he doesn't mention alternating nostrils. This exercise is more akin to what Gheranda calls Bellows (*bhastrika,* see chapter 7).

The Inversion Process (*vyut krama;* 1.57) and the Cooling Process (*sit krama;* 1.58–59) are the reverse of each other: in the former, you sniff water in through the nostrils and spit it out through the mouth; in the latter, you drink water through the mouth and force it out through the nostrils. It's also possible, though Gheranda doesn't mention it, to practice the Inversion Process using just air instead of water. This will be the subject of Practice 2.

For Practice 1, we'll work with a variation of the Air Process practice. Unlike Gheranda, we'll breathe through both nostrils at the same time. Unlike Svatmarama, only the exhalation will be active; the inhalation will be a passive "rebound." This reverses the usual roles of the inhalation and exhalation in the breathing cycle, in which the inhalation is active and the exhalation passive.

Practice: Assisted

There are two ways to practice this version of Skull Brightening: you can use your fisted hands to help pump the breath, which is useful for beginners, or if you're more experienced, you can rely solely on your abdominal muscles.

For the hand-assisted practice, make a fist with one hand, then wrap the other around it. Bring them to your lower belly, closer to the pubic bone than the navel. Start by pressing sharply but lightly up and into (that is, diagonally) your abdomen, aiming in the general direction of your kidneys. This will force air out of your lungs; the amount will depend on how much pressure you apply and how sharply you apply it. Quickly release the pressure on your lower abdomen, which will cause the lungs to passively suck air back in. Repeat this push and release eight to ten times to get the hang of it, working slowly and gently until you determine exactly how much pressure is appropriate for you. Gradually increase the force and speed of the pressure and the number of repetitions. *Stop* right away if you feel light-headed or dizzy, and when you go back to the practice the next time, use less pressure and fewer repetitions.

To start, a reasonable speed for your exhalations is about 1 per second. Gradually increase your speed over the next few weeks of regular practice to about 2 exhalations per second. A reasonable goal is two or three rounds of twenty-five to fifty repetitions each.

Practice: Unassisted

The unassisted practice relies solely on contracting and releasing the lower abdominal muscles. During practice, keep your face and body relaxed and the sound of the exhalation soft.

Traditional Benefit

This exercise balances the bodily humors.

Application

Both exercises in this section can be used to open an asana practice, and Skull Brightening is especially useful as a warm-up for *pranayama* practice.

SECTION 2: EYES

TRATAKA

> *TRATAKA* • an ascetic's method of fixing the eye on one object

There are two kinds of Trataka: external (*bahya*), which is described by both Svatmarama and Gheranda, and internal (*antara*), which we'll come to when we work on Shiva's Seal (*shambhavi mudra*) in chapter 8.

Practice: External Trataka

External Trataka is the soul of simplicity. To paraphrase Gheranda, Without "winking" (*nimesha unmesha*), stare at a small object (or *lakshya*, "mark") until tears begin to fall. It's important here not to "wink" or blink. The object of interest can be something mundane, like the tip of a lighted candle, or spiritually charged, such as an icon of your favorite deity.

Shri Yogendra recommends starting this practice by staring at a candle flame, set no closer to your eyes than 16 inches and no farther than 20 inches, for about 2 minutes at a time. He continues that after a few months, you should switch to staring at light reflected off the surface of clear water in a wide bowl, positioned so that the light is centered in the bowl. This practice should be continued for 3 minutes.

Traditional Benefit

Trataka cures diseases of the eyes and, like Thread Neti (*sutra neti*), confers "divine sight."

Caution: Avoid using a candle if you've been diagnosed with epilepsy, because the flickering light could potentially induce a seizure; instead, focus on a small black dot on a piece of cardboard. People with multiple sclerosis or diabetes should also avoid candle gazing, which can harm their retinas.

Application

This practice is itself a form of meditation and serves well as a preparation for *shambhavi mudra* (see chapter 8).

Little Lamp: Gaze (*Drishti*)

Trataka can be used as a preparation for directed "gaze" (*drishti*), a technique traditionally applied during some asanas (see for example, *padmasana* and *simhasana*) and in meditation. The *Mandala-Brahmana-Upanishad* distinguishes three kinds of *drishti*: that with the eyes closed (*ama*, or "night," the new moon); that with the eyes half-open (*pratipat*, "hasten to," first day of lunar fortnight, half moon); and that with the eyes fully open (*purnima*, "full moon"). There are then two main marks (*lakshyas*) to direct the eyes toward: the tip of the nose (*nasa agra*) and the middle of the forehead (*bhru madhya*). The Upanishad instructs us to gaze at the tip of the nose until we see a deep darkness at the root of the palate. After a while, we'll see a light (*jyotis*) in the form of an endless sphere, which is the Absolute, or Brahman.

SECTION 3: NOSE AND SINUSES

WATER NETI (JALA NETI)

> *JALA* • water
> *NETI* • the drawing of a thread through the nose and mouth

There are two kinds of *neti*: thread (*sutra*), which is described by both Svatmarama and Gheranda; and water (*jala*), which is the more common and accessible type. It involves pouring water through the nasal passages, a practice that understandably repels many students. I admit the idea seems a bit odd at first, but once you get over your initial reluctance, I think you'll find Water Neti to be a most useful exercise, not only as preparation for *pranayama*, but as a simple cleaning out to start your day.

Practice

To practice Water Neti, you'll need what's usually called a *neti* pot, a small vessel with a long, tapering snout that holds about a cup of water. You can find such pots easily nowadays; I just saw one for sale at my local big-box drugstore, and a Google search for "*neti* pot" elicited nearly four hundred thousand hits.

Fill the pot to the brim with body-temperature water and—this is important—about a quarter teaspoon of sea salt. Don't forget the salt; pouring plain water through your sinuses is an unpleasant experience. Stand over a sink or bathtub, and tilt your head sideways (so one ear faces the basin). Insert the snout securely in the upper nostril, press the base of your tongue to the back of your throat to block your esophagus, and tilt the pot upward. The water will immediately pour out of the lower nostril, unless your sinuses are plugged with mucus. In this latter case, you'll have to be patient until the water can dissolve the blockage, which you can help along by wiggling your nose. Eventually the warm water will break through the mucus "dam," and out it will come . . . you'll see. Use a half pot for each nostril, then hold your head straight over the sink and snort the residual water out.

Traditional Benefit

Both Svatmarama and Gheranda teach only Thread Neti, which is supposed to confer "divine sight" (*divya drishti*).

Application

Jala neti is useful both in daily life and as a preparation for *pranayama*. It's a good way to start the day, along with all the usual routines like brushing your teeth and washing your face.

SECTION 4: EARS

EAR CLEANING (KARNA DHAUTI)

KARNA · ear

Practice

Traditionally the tip of the index finger is used to clean out the ear canals. Your doctor would undoubtably advise against this. Modern methods commonly use some kind of solution to flush out the ears.

Traditional Benefit

With constant practice, a yogi will hear the subtle inner sound (*nada*) (see chapter 8).

SECTION 5: TEETH, TONGUE, AND THROAT

CLEANING THE ROOT OF THE TEETH (DANTA MULA DHAUTI)

DANTA · tooth

Practice

The original instruction nowadays is to use an extract called *Acacia catechu* (*khadi*) or clay or fresh earth (*mrittika*) to rub the base or root (*mula*) of the teeth. It turns out the catechu is a strong astringent and antioxidant; it is an ingredient of pan, the betel-leaf preparation widely consumed in India.

Traditional Benefit

Gheranda would be very popular with the American Dental Association. He places particular importance on *danta mula dhauti,* calls the practice "esteemed," and advises us to clean our teeth every morning (*prabhata*).

Tongue Cleaning (Jihva Dhauti)

JIHVA · tongue

Practice

Traditionally this practice, which is also called *jihva shodhana,* was performed by scraping what all of my sources call the "root of the tongue" (*lambika mula*), although *lambika* derives from *lamb,* meaning "to hang down," and refers to the uvula or soft palate, not the tongue) with the joined index, middle, and ring fingers. Today, however, it's best to use the edge of a spoon or a "tongue scraping" tool, which is readily available online. Once the surface of the tongue is scraped clean, Gheranda instructs us to use a pair of tongs to pull the muscle out, rub it with butter, and stretch or "milk" (*doha*) it over and over at sunrise and sunset until it becomes "long" (*dirghata*). Why do we want a long tongue? See chapter 6.

Traditional Benefit

According to Gheranda, this practice can get rid of disease, old age, and death.

Cleaning with a Stick (Danda Dhauti)

DANDA · stick, stalk

Practice

The "stalk" referred to is plantain, turmeric, or cane. This is slipped into the throat and rubbed around to remove phlegm, bile, and mucus (*kleda*).

Cleaning by Vomiting (Vamana Dhauti)

VAMANA · the act of vomiting or ejecting from the mouth; emitting, emission; an emetic; offering oblations to fire

Practice

When we're finished eating, Gheranda says we should drink water until we fill up our throat, then vomit the water. This sounds a bit extreme, so it might be better just to gargle with some warm water.

Traditional Benefit

This practice is supposed to prevent humoral disorders. Cleaning by vomiting is similar to a practice called Elephant Technique (*gaja karani*), described by Svatmarama (*Hatha-Yoga-Pradipika* 2.38).

Section 6: Belly

Fire-Moving Cleaning (Vahni Sara Dhauti)

VAHNI · digestive fire; also "any draft animal; one who conveys or bears along, applied to a charioteer or rider, or to various gods; the conveyer or bearer of oblations to the gods, especially said of Agni, 'fire'"

Practice

Also called *agni sara dhauti,* this exercise is similar to and serves as a preparation for Skull Brightening (*kapala bhati*).

Gheranda tells us to contract the lower belly, or the "navel knot" (*nabhi granthi*), toward the spine one hundred times. It is best to start out with five to ten contractions and gradually increase the number to one hundred over several weeks or months, depending on the regularity of your practice.

Traditional Benefit

This practice is said to cure intestinal diseases and increase digestive fire (*jathara agni*). Gheranda adds that it brings "success" (*siddhi*). Other sources note that it massages the abdominal organs and tones the abdominal muscles.

SECTION 7: MISCELLANEOUS ACTS (FOR INFORMATION ONLY)

AIR-MOVING CLEANING (VATA SARA DHAUTI)

VATA · wind, air

Practice

Shape your lips into Crow Seal (*kaka cancu*; see chapter 6), slowly inhale through the pursed lips, fill the stomach with air, perform Nauli (described later in this chapter), then pass the air out through the anus.

Traditional Benefit

This practice purifies the body (*deha*), destroys "all disease" (*sarva roga*), and augments (*vardha*) the body's digestive fire (*anala*).

WATER-MOVING CLEANING (VARI SARA DHAUTI)

VARI · water

Practice

Fill the throat with water up to the top (*kantha*), move it through the belly, and push it out through the lower passage (a euphemism for the rectum).

Traditional Benefit

This practice cleans the body and makes it "divine" (*deva*).

EXPELLED CLEANING (BAHISH KRITA DHAUTI)

bahis · out, forth, outward

Practice

With Crow's Seal (see chapter 6), fill the stomach with air, hold for 90 minutes, then move the air through the intestines and out the anus. Next, stand (or squat in Superior Pose; see chapter 5) in navel-deep water, draw out your long intestine (*shakti nadi*), wash it clean, and push it back inside your belly. This practice is difficult even for the gods to obtain (*durlabha*).

Traditional Benefit

This practice creates a divine body.

Cleaning with a Cloth (Vaso Dhauti)

VASAS · cloth

Practice

This practice involves swallowing a long, thin cloth and performing Nauli. After the cloth has fully swabbed your stomach, you pull it out.

Traditional Benefit

Cloth is a fix-all for a variety of conditions: an abdominal tumor (*gulma*), fever, diseases of the spleen (*plihan*), leprosy (*kushtha*), and humoral disorders. Svatmarama calls this practice *dhauti karman* and notes that it cures coughing, asthma, an enlarged spleen, leprosy, and a variety of humoral diseases.

Root Purifying (Mula Shodhana)

Practice

The "root" being cleaned here is the rectum, washed either with a stick of tumeric (which supposedly has antiseptic qualities) or a handy digit.

Traditional Benefit

This practice prevents intestinal problems, stokes the digestive fire (*vahni*), and confers beauty (*kanti*) and health (*pushti*).

WET BLADDER (JALA VASTI)

VASTI · bladder, abdomen

Practice

Squat in navel-deep water (in Superior Pose) with a special pipe inserted in the anus, then contract and dilate the anal sphincter.

Traditional Benefit

The wet practice prevents urinary diseases (*prameha*), bowel diseases (*udavarta*), and problems with "cruel wind" (*krura vayu*). The practitioner gets a body like the god of love (Kama, the Hindu Cupid). Svatmarama adds that this exercise cures enlargement of the spleen (*gulma*) and abdomen (*udara*); clears and brightens (*prasada*) the mind and senses; stokes the digestive fire; and eliminates defects (*dosha*).

DRY BLADDER (SHUSHKA VASTI)

SHUSHKA · dry, arid

Practice

This practice is also called *sthala vasti*. Sit in Intense-Stretch-of-the-West Pose (*pashchima uttanasana*; see chapter 5). Move the belly (*vasti cala*) and contract and dilate the anus with the Dawn Horse Seal (*ashvini mudra*; see chapter 6).

Traditional Benefit

This prevents intestinal disorders, stokes the digestive fire (*jathara agni*), and cures flatulence (*amavata*).

NAULI

Practice

Rotate the stomach quickly like a "whirlpool" (*avarta*). Svatmarama praises Nauli as the "crown" or "top-knot" (*mauli*) of Hatha practices.

Traditional Benefit

This exercise, which is also called *lauli* (from *lauliki,* or "rolling"), cures all diseases and stokes the digestive fire. It always brings happiness (*ananda*) and dries up all defects and diseases (*dosha*).

TURN OUT THE LIGHT

Nowadays our yoga practice seems isolated from our daily life. But many of these simple housecleaning exercises — like brushing our teeth and cleaning our ears — remind us how intimately connected life and practice were for the old yogis. Everything they did, even the most mundane chores, somehow related to their practice and fed into the larger effort toward self-understanding, like small streams combining into a great river.

4

ASANA THROUGH
THE AGES

A S A N A · sitting, sitting down; sitting
in peculiar posture according to the custom of
devotees; the manner of sitting forming part of the
eightfold observances of ascetics; halting, stopping,
encamping; abiding, dwelling; seat, place, stool; the
withers of an elephant, the part where the driver
sits; maintaining a post against an enemy . . .
— "Asana," freely adapted from the *Sanskrit-English
Dictionary* by Monier Monier-Williams, 159

JUST AS WE CAN WRITE a history of yoga, we can do the same for asana. I suspect that many yoga students today would define the word *asana* as either "pose" or "posture" and say that this particular practice has been pretty much the same for thousands of years. But *asana* literally means "seat" or "stool," derived from the verb *as*, "to sit." It's really a relic of distant past (at least twenty-five hundred years ago) when an asana wasn't a pose at all but a platform or "steady seat" (*sthiram asanam*) where the yogi sat to meditate. The elements of this asana platform were dictated by tradition. According to the third- or fourth-century B.C.E. *Bhagavad-Gita* (6.11), it should be erected in a clean place, neither too high nor too low, and covered with a special kind of grass, a cloth, and the hide of a deer or tiger. There were practical considerations for all of these directions. Since he meditated out of doors and was exposed to the elements, the yogi needed a platform high enough to raise him off the ground, which might be wet or cold or creeping with creepy things, but not so high that a misstep would send him tumbling disastrously head over heels. (I'm using masculine pronouns here because back then yoga practitioners were almost entirely male. The feminine equivalents will get equal play later on.) The grass, cloth, and skin padded his bottom during what were probably long sitting meditation sessions. There's no indication that, in those far-off days, there were more than a handful of poses in the yogi's repertoire, all of them sitting, the most enduring of which is Lotus Pose. What follows is a brief history of asana, beginning with the first systematic presentation of a yoga practice, Patanjali's *Yoga-Sutra*, dated 200 C.E.

PATANJALI: THE *YOGA-SUTRA* (200 C.E.)

Around the time Patanjali (or some anonymous yogi who credited Patanjali) compiled the *Yoga-Sutra*, the meaning of *asana* had expanded to include both the platform and, as we understand it today, the yogi's physical pose. The latter was still essentially a "seat" or sitting pose, since it's likely that Patanjali thought of an asana as a meditative pose. He doesn't specify any poses, because the *Yoga-Sutra* is an outline of his system and not an instructional manual. But he does note that whatever the sitting pose, it must meet two essential criteria to qualify as an asana (*Yoga-Sutra* 2.46): it must be "firm, solid, motionless, still, calm" (*sthira*), and at the same time, it must be "comfortable" (*sukha*). Notice that Patanjali's "firm and comfortable" echoes the directions for a well-built asana platform, which was supposed to be "steady" and not too high or too low, but comfortably just right. It's as if the yogi's physical body assumed the role and qualities of his supporting seat.

Notice too that Patanjali is looking for balance between rigidity on the one hand and flaccidity on the other. Why are firmness and comfort so important? The yogi needs to sit firmly because fidgeting distracts from the intense concentration needed for meditation; at the same time, he needs to be comfortable because he'll presumably be sitting in one place for a long time, and being firm but uncomfortable is just as distracting as being comfortable but antsy. Looking to the *Gita* (6.13) again, this delicate balancing act between the two extremes is achieved, Krishna says, when the sitter's head, neck, and torso are *sama*, a word that means "even, same, equal, neutral, equally distant from extremes, straight, honest; easy; full, complete, whole, entire; equanimous, imperturbable." It's interesting that the word Krishna uses for physical alignment also implies psychological alignment, suggesting that the former naturally leads to the latter and that this way of sitting, in and of itself, is actually a form of meditation.

The proposition that physical alignment is the foundation, not only of a successful asana practice, but of yoga practice in general, is widely accepted today. The progenitor, or at least the main proponent, of this idea — and himself a master of alignment — is B. K. S. Iyengar. Over the last sixty years or so, Iyengar has developed and refined principles of alignment to a sophisticated degree. His way of describing the two aspects of asana, which he calls posing and reposing, seems much akin to Patanjali's firm and comfortable:

> Posing means action . . . assuming a fixed position of limbs and body as represented by the particular asana being performed. Reposing means reflection on the pose . . . re-thought and re-adjusted so that the various limbs and parts of the body are positioned in their places in a proper order and feel rested and soothed, and the mind experiences the tranquility and calmness of bones, joints, muscles, fibres and cells.[1]

So while Iyengar is rightly recognized and acknowledged today for his revolutionary work with alignment in asana, the germ of the idea can be traced back more than two thousand years to books like the *Gita* and the *Shvetashvatara-Upanishad* (White Horse Upanishad; 2.8, translation by Patrick Olivelle):

> When he keeps his body straight, with the three sections [i.e., torso, neck, and head] erect, and draws the senses together with the mind into his heart, a wise man shall cross all the frightful rivers with the boat consisting of . . . brahman.

LITTLE LAMP: THERE ARE MORE WAYS THAN ONE TO SKIN AN ASANA

Most students and teachers nowadays accept the "steady and comfortable" criteria without question as the *only* way to perform asana. But as my friend Stu Sovatsky writes in his book *Words from the Soul*, there's likely another approach that greatly predates Patanjali's focus on the straightened spine. Sovatsky sees the "straight-back path" as an intentional "taming" or rigidification of the "originary emergence" of spontaneous asanas, which were expressed through "yearning, quaking, shaking, davening, throbbing, swaying."[2] This Dionysian approach—as opposed to Iyengar's Apollonian—is most beautifully expressed today in the teaching of a pair of extraordinary yogis, Victor van Kooten and Angela Farmer.

VYASA: THE *YOGA BHASHYA* (400 C.E.)

It's not clear—at least, not to me—if there were other kinds of asanas besides the sitting variety being practiced in Patanjali's time. It's likely there were, but most of them didn't look anything like the ones we practice today. Let's jump ahead two to three hundred years and look in the oldest surviving commentary or "discussion" (*bhashya*) on the *Yoga-Sutra*, written by (or at least attributed to) someone named Vyasa, the Arranger. In his remarks on sutra 2.46, which is the famous dictum *sthira-sukham-asanam* mentioned earlier, he names eleven asanas, most of which, like Lotus and Hero, are still sitting meditative poses. But at least three—Elephant, Camel, and Curlew (or Heron)—are plainly different. Swami Kuvalayananda writes that these poses cultivate "physiological advantages," by which he means the health of the nervous and endocrine systems, "because through these two systems the health of the whole human organism can be secured."[3]

Where did these early poses come from? The names strongly suggest that they're human imitations of the seats, or poses, of common (for India) living creatures. A later commentator on Patanjali, Vachaspati Mishra in the mid-ninth century, says as much: "The Curlew and the other seats may be understood by actually seeing a curlew and the other animals seated" (translation by James Woods). What did these poses look like? Camel Pose is a familiar backbend, which we'll practice in Section 6, though its traditional form is much different from its modern incarnation. Curlew or Heron (*kraunchasana*), is also a well-known modern pose, although no one seems to know what the traditional form looked like. And Elephant Pose (*gajasana*)? It might have looked as described in the nineteenth-century *Shri-Tattva-Nidhi*:

> Lie on the stomach. Place the toes and the palms . . . on the floor, raise the buttocks and let the head hang down between the arms, the nose on the ground where the navel was originally. Bring the nose forward as far as the palms . . . This should be repeated again and again.[4]

TIRUMULAR: THE *TIRU MANTIRAM* (700 C.E.)

However many asanas there were in Vyasa's time—and there's a hint in the *bhashya* that there were more than the eleven he names—they still take a backseat to meditation in yoga practice. Asanas were a preliminary step, and the situation didn't change much for many centuries. For example, there's the south Indian book honored as the Tamil Veda, the *Tiru Mantiram* (Holy Mantra), written by the poet-sage Tirumular around 700 C.E. Of the 3,047 verses in the book, only six—that's right, *six*—are dedicated to a perfunctory description of eight (or nine, it isn't clear) asanas, all but one of which are sitting.

GORAKSHA: THE *GORAKSHA-SHATAKA* (1200 C.E.)

The sea change in the number, role, and status of asanas makes an early appearance around 1200 in the *Goraksha-Shataka*, or "Goraksha's One Hundred [Verses]" (*shataka* means "consisting of a hundred," though the book actually has 101 verses), attributed to the semilegendary teacher Goraksha. Here we enter the realm of Hatha Yoga in one of the school's oldest surviving books. Meditation is still central to this school's practice, but it now shares the limelight with asana, *pranayama*, and mudra. In 300 B.C.E., an asana was a raised platform; five hundred years later, the word reached out to embrace the yogi's physical sitting pose; and two hundred years after that, we have the names of eleven asanas, a few of which may have some undefined function other than simply supplying a seat for meditation.

Then sometime in the three hundred years between the emergence of Hatha in 900 C.E. and the appearance of the *Goraksha-Shataka*, there's a veritable explosion of asanas to the tune, you might remember, of 8.4 million. Be that as it may, the author of the *Goraksha-Shataka* (which is attributed to Goraksha, though there's no proof he wrote it or even existed) includes just two: Lotus Pose (which he calls *kamalasana; kamala* being another name for "lotus") and Perfected Pose (*siddhasana*).

SVATMARAMA YOGENDRA:
THE *HATHA-YOGA-PRADIPIKA* (1350 C.E.)

Our next stop is our first sourcebook, Svatmarama's *Hatha-Yoga-Pradipika* (Light on the Forceful Union-Method; or *Hatha-Pradipika*, as some would have it), which we encountered a while back in this book's introduction. Svatmarama, a practical-minded fellow, says nothing about 8.4 million asanas, only the eighty-four taught by Shiva (*Hatha-Yoga-Pradipika* 1.33). Of the fifteen asanas he describes, about half might be considered meditative poses, though even at this relatively late date, three of the four that he considers the best of the lot — Perfected, Lotus, and Fortunate (*bhadrasana*) — are still of this variety. The rest — like Peacock (*mayurasana*), Bow (*dhanurasana*), and Rooster (*kukkutasana*) — can be considered physiological asanas that are said to calm the mind, stimulate the appetite, and ward off disease — among other things.

Here's a quality of asana we haven't run across before in the older books, though no doubt it was around before 1350, maybe as far back as Vyasa. Many asanas, in addition to being meditative seats, are now credited (at times, perhaps exaggeratedly so) with extraordinary preventive, stimulating, and healing powers. We can readily understand and agree with the idea that a regular asana practice will help us ward

off disease and maybe lead a healthier and longer life, but who believes — and is willing to test the veracity of — the claim that through
the practice of Peacock Pose we can digest the deadliest poison in the
world (see *Hatha-Yoga-Pradipika* 1.31)? It's noted that only the "wise"
(*dhimat*) can tap into the potential of Lotus, suggesting that there's
more to an asana than meets the eye, that it won't supply us with its full
benefit unless a certain intensity of insight is reached and applied to its
performance.

Asana now steps fully into its second role. Depending on the asana,
it can be a seat for the meditating yogi; it can be a preparation for that
seat; or it can serve both functions, blurring the line between meditative and physical asanas. More than eight hundred years earlier, Patanjali (in *Yoga-Sutra* 1.30) recognized sickness (*vyadhi*) as the first of
nine obstacles to practice. It makes sense that sitting in the prescribed
manner might not be so easy if you have a cold or indigestion. While
he offers eight ways to counteract the obstacles, none of them involve
asana. The conviction that asanas have therapeutic value is, like the
importance of alignment, widely accepted today. But as we saw with
alignment, the rapidly growing industry of yoga therapy has ancient
roots. Please note that in the practice chapters of this book, I give the
traditional benefits, if I can find any, for each asana, mudra, *pranayama,*
or meditation — not what we moderns believe are its health advantages. To find the latter, I recommend *Light on Yoga,* with the understanding that what Iyengar says is mostly anecdotal; only recently
have researchers started looking into the health benefits of Hatha Yoga
using Western "scientific" standards.

YOGA UPANISHADS (CA. 1400 C.E.)

Around the same time as the *Hatha-Yoga-Pradipika* was written, there
appeared a loose collection of about twenty short books known as the
Yoga Upanishads. None of the dozen or so I have access to say anything
about the 8.4 million or even eighty-four asanas. Many of them only
mention a handful, and typically they're sitting poses. For example, the
Varaha-Upanishad (Boar Upanishad) names eleven asanas, only two of
which — Peacock and Rooster — are definitely physiological poses. But

in a few of these books, we encounter a suggestion that ultimately an asana is neither a platform nor a pose but a particular configuration of consciousness. The *Mandala-Brahmana-Upanishad* says that "being firm in the unshaken spiritual wisdom constitutes asana." The *Tejo-Bindu-Upanishad* (Radiance Point Upanishad) puts it like this:

> There is silence in children, but with words latent; whereas the knowers of Brahman have it (silence) but without words. That should be known as the "lonely seat" in which there is no man in the beginning, middle, or end, and through which all this (universe) is fully pervaded. The illusion of Brahma and all other beings takes place within one twinkling (of His eye). That should be known as asana . . . in which one has with ease and without fatigue (uninterrupted) meditation on Brahman . . . that is endless bliss and that is second less [i.e., that drives away all worldly pleasures]. That is called siddhasana . . . in which the siddhas (psychical personages) have succeeded in realizing the endless One as the support of the universe . . .[5]

SECRECY IN THE *SHIVA-SAMHITA* AND *GHERANDA-SAMHITA*

The praise for the power of asana we began to hear with Svatmarama gets louder and more miraculous with Anonymous/Shiva. Merely by *thinking* of *siddhasana*, for example, the yogi is freed from evil-mindedness (*papa; Shiva-Samhita* 3.101); through *svastikasana*, he destroys "all suffering" (*sarva duhkha; Shiva-Samhita* 3.115). It's no wonder, given the potential for misuse and abuse of the asanas in the wrong hands, that Shiva exhorts us time and again to keep the asanas "secret" (*guhya; Shiva-Samhita* 3.101, 3.115) or "preserved, protected, concealed" (*gopaniya; Shiva-Samhita* 3.112).

TURN OUT THE LIGHT

Whereas the *Shiva-Samhita* is blue-sky philosophical, the *Gheranda-Samhita* is down-to-earth practical. Anonymous/Gheranda mentions that among the 8.4 million ananas, eighty-four are chief or best (*vish-ishta*). While Goraksha focused on only two, Svatmarama fifteen, and Shiva four of the eighty-four, Gheranda settles on the thirty-two he believes are most "agreeable, suitable, useful" (*shubha*) for human consumption. These poses are the subject of the next chapter.

5

GHERANDA'S
THIRTY-TWO ASANAS:
A PRACTICE OVERVIEW

WHAT ARE THE thirty-two most useful asanas? Here's the list in their original Gheranda order (see pp. 80–81). The first column on the left shows the verse number(s) in chapter 2 of the *Gheranda-Samhita*. Next comes the English translation of the pose followed by its Sanskrit name in italics (remember that technically there aren't any capitals in Sanskrit, so all the pose names are in lowercase letters). The third column shows the Iyengar equivalent (if any), and the last two columns indicate which of the poses are also found in the *Hatha-Yoga-Pradipika* and *Shiva-Samhita* and where. I've marked the seven asanas in which a specific gaze (*drishti*) is performed: five at the tip of the nose (*nasa agra drishti*) with a downward-pointing triangle, and two at the midbrow (*bhru madhya drishti*) with an upward-pointing triangle (we'll go into *drishtis* in chapter 6). Finally, what I'm calling the Net-Bearing Bond (*jalandhara bandha*) is applied in five poses, which are marked with a circle.

GENERAL CHARACTERISTICS

What can we say in general about the thirty-two asanas? Some obvious things leap right off the page (or would if the pose descriptions were included in the chart). Almost half are named after living creatures, a tradition that stretches back at least to Vyasa twelve hundred years ago. There are four mammals (Lion, Camel, Bull, and Cow); two birds (Rooster

78

and Peacock); two reptiles (Serpent and Tortoise—and one Tortoise variation); a fish (Fish); an amphibian (Frog—with one Frog variation); an insect (Locust); and two mythic creatures, a sea monster (Makara) and a humanoid eagle (Garuda). To this group, we could technically add five more:

- Lord of Fish, which honors the first human Hatha teacher, Matsyendra, who in some versions of his story began his life as an actual fish
- Cowherd, which honors Matsyendra's prize pupil, Goraksha
- Hero, presumably a human
- Tree and Lotus, which while not exactly "creatures" are nonetheless living things

Again we see the close relationship between asana and the natural world. It doesn't seem far-fetched to imagine that the world itself is ensouled and practicing yoga; that it, too, is searching for its authentic self; and that humans are playing along, matching the world's asanas.

About half the poses are sitting poses, which tells us that despite the enormous jump in the number of asanas since Patanjali's time, they still play second fiddle to sitting meditation (and *pranayama*) in Hatha Yoga. It was not until the twentieth century that asana stepped into a starring role. We also see that five of the sitting poses—Perfected, Freedom, Fortunate, Secret, and Cowherd—are so closely related as to be almost indistinguishable. I'll go into details about this in Section 11.

There are ten or so asanas that probably weren't a challenge for the old Indian yogis but will likely give the average twenty-first-century Westerner some degree of trouble. This points to a basic cultural difference between us and India: our habitual chair-sitting often results in tight hips and groins, while Indians' crossed-leg floor-sitting or squatting helps keeps their hips and groins open. The main troublemaker here is one of the quintessential Hatha asanas, Lotus Pose, aided and abetted by its six companions among the thirty-two—Hero, Fish, Lord of Fish, Rooster, Raised Tortoise, and Yoga Pose—that involve either a full or half-leg lock. Many of us dream of experiencing the "yogic-ness" of sitting in this pose, but realistically, if we value our knees, we should avoid this pose like the plague until we've done some serious preparation to release our cemented hips and groins.

Verse(s) in chapter 2 of *Gheranda-Samhita*	English *(Sanskrit)*	Iyengar Equivalent	Verse(s) in chapter 1 of *Hatha-Yoga-Pradipika*	Verse(s) in chapter 3 of *Shiva-Samhita*
7	Perfected *(siddha)* ▲ ●	Same	35–43	97–101
8	Lotus *(padma)* ▼ ●	Same	44–49	102–107
9–10	Fortunate *(bhadra)* ▼ ●	Bound Angle Pose *baddha konasana*	53–54	
11	Freedom *(mukta)*	None		
12	Diamond *(vajra)*	Similar to *virasana*		
13	Auspicious *(svastika)*	None	19	113–115
14–15	Lion *(simha)* ▼ ●	Same	50–52	
16	Cow Face *(gomukha)*	Same	20	
17	Hero *(vira)*	Leg position for *bharadvajasana* II		21
18	Bow *(dhanu)*	Same	25 (different pose)	
19	Death *(mrita)* (or Corpse, *shava*)	Same	32	
20	Secret *(gupta)*	None		
21	Fish *(matsya)*	Same		
22–23	Lord of Fish *(matsyendra)* ▲	*ardha matsyendrasana* I	26–27	
24–25	Cowherd *(goraksha)* ▼ ●	None (same name, different pose)	28–29	108–112
26	Intense-Stretch-of-West *(pashchimottana)*	Same		

27	Superior (*utkata*)	Similar (see also GS 1.45–46)	
28	Contracted (*sankata*)	Leg Position for *gomukhasana*	
29–30	Peacock (*mayura*)	Same	30–31
31	Rooster (*kukkuta*)	Same	23
32	Tortoise (*kurma*)	None (same name, different pose)	22
33	Raised Tortoise (*uttana kurma*)	Similar to *garbha pindasana*	24
34	Frog (*manduka*)	None	
35	Raised Frog (*uttana manduca*)	None	
36	Tree (*vriksha*)	Same	
37	Eagle (*garuda*)	None (same name, different pose)	
38	Bull (*trisha*)	None	
39	Locust (*shalabha*)	Similar, hand position different	
40	Sea Monster (*makara*)	Similar, but more of a back bend	
41	Camel (*ushtra*)	None, similar to *dhanurasana* (modern version)	
42–43	Serpent (*bhujanga*)	Same	
44–45	Union-Method (*yoga*) ▼	Similar	

▼ Gaze at the tip of the nose (*nasa agra drishti*)
● Perform Net-Bearing Bond (*jalandhara bandha*)
▲ Gaze at the mid-brow (*bhru madhya drishti*)

We don't have to look far to find a clear example of what a typical Indian thinks of Lotus. Look at the pose (#45) in Iyengar's *Light on Yoga*. Each of the two hundred poses in the book is assigned a kind of "intensity index" on a scale from 1 to 60, with 1 (like *tadasana*, #1) being the easiest and 60 (like *triang mukhottanasana*, literally, the intense stretch of the three limbs, i.e., arms, legs, and torso, #198) the most challenging. For the average Westerner, based on some of the other poses and their ratings, we might rank Lotus in the high teens or low twenties, but Iyengar gives it a 4; for comparison's sake, the far more accessible (for us) sitting poses Intense-Stretch-of-the-West (*pashchima uttanasana*) and Seated Angle (*upavishtha konasana*) are rated at 6 and 9. (It would be interesting to know how Iyengar would rate Lotus today, since in 1966 when *Light on Yoga* was first published, he was far less familiar with Western students).

But the Lotus-type poses are the only ones that expose the gulf between Western and Indian lower extremities. Our tendency toward tight hips and groins is no secret, but what isn't as well known is that we have a similar tendency toward tight ankles. We can lay this condition at the feet, so to speak, of constantly wearing shoes, which binds our ankles like a cast; we also mostly walk on hard, level surfaces that don't put our ankles through their full paces. We'll find out firsthand, or maybe "first-foot," about our tight ankles when we get to traditional Tortoise Pose, which requires us to sit with our feet everted, that is, turned out so the inner edges rest on the floor.

THE ORIGINAL YOGA PROJECT

What really catches the eye of a dyed-in-the-wool (though not certified) Iyengarite of the early twenty-first century is Gheranda's disturbingly haphazard presentation. Scanning this list many years ago, it occurred to me that it would be possible to arrange the thirty-two asanas in some kind of coherent order that would firstly make the more challenging ones more accessible and secondly make each one more efficacious.

As soon as I set about this project, which I dubbed Homage to the Source and which we've renamed Original Yoga for this book, I ran into several roadblocks. First I bumped up against the near sameness of the five poses in what I called the Perfected Family (see Section 11). I realized that it wouldn't be useful (or, more to the point, very interesting) to put all of them in the sequence. So risking an insult to tradition, I kept one (Perfected), changed one slightly to use as a Lotus preparation (Auspicious), and dropped three altogether (Freedom, Secret, and Cowherd). This left me with twenty-nine asanas. Next I was brought up short by a similar problem with three more pairs of poses: Yoga Pose is the same as Lotus except for its hand position; Eagle Pose is a spread-out version of Tortoise; and Contracted Pose is an intensified version of Cow Face. Also, Eagle and Contracted are both well-nigh impossible for the average Western student. So into the figurative storage trunk with the three Perfected Family members went Yoga, Eagle, and Contracted; I was down to twenty-six poses. Finally there was the major hurdle of the six Lotus Family poses. If I banished most or all of them, there wouldn't be much of a sequence left, so in the end, I decided to keep five and excise only Raised Tortoise, which seemed particularly unfriendly to Westerners.

The question I asked myself at this point was, do I sequence just the twenty-five survivors, or do I stay somewhat true to tradition—I did, after all, just banish seven poses with a wave of my magic wand—and try to find replacements to bring the sequence back to thirty-two asanas? I decided that, for whatever reason, Gheranda wanted thirty-two, and I should at least respect that number. But where would I find the seven fill-ins?

One arrived in the form of the Bow Pose. Happily for me, if we compare Svatmarama's version with Gheranda's, we find that the same name is used for two different poses—a not-unheard-of-situation with the old books, where standardization is somewhat lacking. In the *Hatha-Yoga-Pradipika,* Bow Pose is a forward bend (today we call it *akarna dhanurasana*), but it is a backbend (as we know it today) in the *Gheranda-Samhita.* The other six I found in Gheranda's fourth chapter on the mudras, which we'll work with primarily in chapter 6. Five mudras among the twenty-five described are, if not asanas in fact, then at least very asana-like in spirit. They include Pond Seal (*tadagi mudra*); the Bird Catcher Seal (*pashini mudra,* slightly modified here); Great Seal (*maha mudra,* which we'll interpret as Head-to-Knee Pose, or *janu shirshasana*); the Vajroli Seal (left untranslated); and Inverted Action Seal (*viparita karani mudra*).

If you've been reading carefully—and I hope you have been—you'll have noticed that I needed six exercises to get back to thirty-two but named only five Gheranda mudras. Once again, this time thanks to the vagueness of the instructions, the Inverted Action Seal can be interpreted in two ways: as what we call Headstand (*shirshasana*), or as what we call Shoulderstand (*sarvangasana*).

THE ORIGINAL SEQUENCE

So after a good deal of clipping and modifying and stretching the limits of the acceptable, I filled out my thirty-two slots with what I hope is a useful and enjoyable sequence of poses. The following is a brief overview of the Original Yoga sequence, broken down into twelve sections.

Section 1: General Warm-up
  Pond Seal → Bird Catcher Seal
Section 2. Lotus Warm-Up 1
  Diamond Pose → Lion Pose → Frog Pose → Raised Frog
  Pose → Tortoise Pose (Eagle)
Section 3: Lotus Warm-Up 2
  Fortunate Pose → Bull Pose
Section 4: Lotus Poses
  Auspicious Pose → Cow Face Pose (Contracted) → Hero
  Pose → Lotus Pose (Yoga) → Rooster Pose → Fish Pose
  (Raised Tortoise)
Section 5: Forward Bends
  Great Seal → Intense-Stretch-of-the-West Pose → Bow Pose 1
  (Svatmarama's version) → Lord of Fish Pose
Section 6: Backbends
  Sea Monster Pose → Serpent Pose → Locust Pose → Bow
  Pose 2 (Gheranda's version) → Camel Pose
Section 7: Standing Poses
  Superior Pose → Tree Pose
Section 8: Inversion 1
  Inverse Action Seal 1 (Headstand)

Section 9: Abdominal Strengtheners
    Peacock Pose → Vajroli Seal
Section 10: Inversion 2
    Inverse Action Seal 2 (Shoulderstand)
Section 11: Perfected Family
    Auspicious Pose → Cowherd Pose → Secret Pose → Free-
        dom Pose → Perfected Pose
Section 12: Relaxation
    Corpse Pose

You'll notice some parenthesized words in the sequence. Four of them — Eagle, Contracted, Yoga, and Raised Tortoise — are poses that were left out because they were either too similar to another pose (Yoga) or too difficult for a general audience (the other three). However, some students out there might be able to more or less perform or at least like to try these poses, so I've included them as variations in the sequence (I've also omitted the traditional names of these variations to avoid confusion). You can try them or not as you please. Three other left-out poses — Goraksha, Secret, Freedom — will be offered as variations to Perfected Pose in Section 11.

The poses in Sections 2 through 7 of the sequence can be linked together in what we call a *vinyasa* (literally "putting together," or more loosely interpreted "flow"). If you prefer, the poses can be performed without any connecting links — that is, separately, one at a time. I'll describe the poses individually as we go through the following sections, then I'll show how to turn them into a *vinyasa* in Appendix 1.

Traditional Benefits

In keeping with the tenor of this book, I'll only be listing the traditional benefits (if any are are known) for the poses. For the most part, these benefits won't be the usual accolades we read in modern books, and some will seem downright strange. Generally the traditional benefits of asana are the steadiness (*sthairya*), health (*arogya*), and lightness (*laghava*) produced in the body (*Hatha-Yoga-Pradipika* 1.17), that we may assume is mirrored in consciousness. Gheranda tells us that asana brings success (*siddhi*) in the world of mortals (*martya loka*, "who or what must die"; *Gheranda-Samhita* 2.6), though he doesn't define what he means by success. *Hatha-Tatva-Kaumudi* makes the point that the benefits of asana can't be achieved by asana alone, that for it to be effective it must be practiced within the context of other traditional limbs. Sundara Deva writes, "A yogi who is well balanced . . . can alleviate the chronic and *incurable* [italics are mine] diseases and toxicity through the practice of yama, niyama, and asana" (7.4).

General Caution

Original Yoga isn't an advanced sequence, but it's not a beginning one either. Almost every pose has its own potential pitfalls, great or small, but two in particular in the Original sequence need special attention—Lotus and Headstand. If you're not familiar with these exercises, you should ideally have some personal instruction in their finer points from an experienced teacher to supplement the instruction in this book. It's not advisable to practice full Lotus or freestanding Headstand based on what you read in a book, even one as expertly written as this one. I'll give beginners alternatives to work with when we come to these poses, and it's my fervent hope that if you fall into that category, you'll follow my instructions and not strike off into unknown territory on your own. But even if you have some experience with Lotus, you should first warm up carefully with Sections 1 through 3.

SECTION 1. GENERAL WARM-UP

Both of the exercises in this section are taken from the mudra chapter of *Gheranda-Samhita,* and both are practiced while lying supine (face up).

POND SEAL (TADAGI MUDRA)

> *TADAGA* · pond
> *MUDRA* · seal (see chapter 6)

Though Gheranda doesn't specify any particular position, Pond Seal can be done lying supine, in a sitting forward bend, or standing. All he does say is to draw the belly back (*pashchima*) and up (*uttana*)—that is, diagonally—into the torso toward the diaphragm. We'll practice it in the reclining position, face up with the arms stretched overhead along the floor.

This exercise is named after the concave or shallow pondlike shape the belly assumes in the stretch. Although Gheranda suggests that this shape is created muscularly, we'll rely on the belly's natural "energetic" response to the lengthening of the body to make it hollow. If you have one, lay a sandbag an arm's length above your head as you lie on the floor.

Practice

Lie on your back with your knees bent, feet on the floor, heels a foot or so from your buttocks. Inhale your arms straight up toward the ceiling, perpendicular to the floor. First draw the heads of the upper arm bones (the humeri) *down* into the shoulder sockets. This will feel odd initially, because in reaching for the ceiling, the tendency is to reach *from* the shoulder joints. But ideally the humerus heads should be sucked deep into their sockets, and the reach of the arms rooted in the mid-back between the shoulder blades. With your arms still raised vertically, rock slowly side to side, widening the sides of your back torso away from the spine and imagining the reach of the arms coming out of the spine. Inhale and swing your arms overhead, sliding your palms and wrists under the sandbag (if you're using one). Push your feet lightly against the floor and feel how that slides your back torso down, away from your ears and toward your tailbone. As the back torso continues to descend, straighten your arms as much as possible and slide the bag away from the top of your head. Spread your palms beneath the weight of the bag

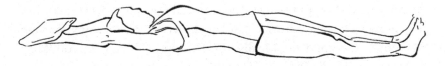

Fig. 1. Pond Seal (*tadagi mudra*).

and imagine the sympathy between them and your shoulder blades. As you open the right palm, the right shoulder blade should follow its lead and spread across your back, and the same with the left palm and shoulder blade.

Now inhale and straighten your right knee, but hold the heel and the back of the leg slightly off the floor. Reach actively down from the back of the pelvis, through the tailbone, along the back of the leg, and out through the heel. Now rotate the thigh inward, so that the toes point slightly to the left. Be sure to turn from the hip joint and not just the ankle. Maintain the reach through the heel and the inner rotation of the thigh, and press the back of the leg down firmly on the floor. Repeat with the left leg. Feel how the inward rotation of the hip joints narrows the front of your pelvis, bringing the two hip points closer to the navel.

Continue to release the back of your pelvis down through your tailbone and out through your heels. In response to this, lift the *back* ribs (keep the front ribs down in the torso) and lengthen through your arms, inching the bag a bit farther away from your head. Now alternate your awareness between the two extremes of your body, reaching first through the heels and then through the arms.

Before we get to the "pond," let me make a couple of points about the belly. Most beginning students think of the belly as a flat sheet between the pubis below and the lower ribs above. But in fact the belly is shaped more like an egg; it sits in the pelvis like an egg in an eggcup. In this image, the perineum — the fleshy base of your pelvis — is the "floor" of your belly, and the diaphragm is its "roof." This means that along with your front belly, there's also a left-side and right-side belly, and a back belly. For convenience, we divide the belly at the navel into halves, so there's a lower belly and an upper belly.

Now I'll ask you to lift your belly. To do that, first fix the pelvis by pinning your tailbone to the floor. Pretend you can lift the egg out of the egg cup, that is, lift the *lower* belly out of the pelvis. As you do this, keep pressing through the heels in one direction and reaching through the arms in the opposite. Ideally, three things will happen: you'll feel the lower front belly "hollow" into the torso, assuming the pond shape (assisted by the continued narrowing of the hip points). Along with this, you'll feel the side bellies narrowing, becoming "waspish"; and finally, you'll feel the perineum, or belly floor, sucked up into the torso and hollowing like the lower belly. Remember that both of these hollowings are an "energetic" response to the length you're creating through your body; they are not created by muscular contraction. The hollow belly is a precursor to the Flying-Up Bond (*uddiyana bandha*) and the hollow perineum to Root Bond (*mula bandha*), both of which are described in chapter 6.

Notice too how the inner and outer muscles (pectoralis major and latissimus dorsi, respectively) of each armpit lengthens as the armpit itself lengthens, narrows, and deepens, creating a pair of smaller ponds. Stay in this stretch anywhere from 2 to 3 minutes, then release the arms and, with an exhalation, draw the thighs into the belly. Wrap your arms around your shins (or the back of your thighs) in what's called Wind-Freeing Pose (*pavana muktasana*). Rock slowly and gently from side to side, again widening the back of your torso as you do. Now set your feet back on the floor for the next pose in this sequence.

LITTLE LAMP: TIMING IN ASANA

As we go through the sequence, you'll see that I suggest a range of time to hold each pose. It's useful to time your stay in the pose for a couple of reasons. First of all, you want to introduce a measure of consistency into your practice. Second, when you're ready to increase your stay in a pose, you want to do it in bite-sized bits and not big chunks of time. If you're comfortable in a pose for, say, 30 seconds, then you should increase by about 15 to 20 seconds and practice at that level for a reasonable length of time before adding another quarter minute. Always remember: progress slowly. As Svatmarama says in regard to *pranayama* (and applies to all the practices), tame the breath slowly, just as a lion (*simha*), elephant (*gaja*), or tiger (*vyaghra*) is tamed slowly, or the practice "hurts, obstructs, kills" (*hanti*) the yogi.

If timing really doesn't appeal to you, then you don't need to time all the poses, but I still highly recommend that you always time any pose involving full or Half-Lotus, as well as Headstand and Shoulderstand. The only pose you needn't time, if you have an open-ended amount of time for practice, is Corpse Pose — unless you tend to shortchange your stay in the pose. The rule of thumb for Corpse is the 5-to-1 rule: for every 5 minutes you practice, you should stay in Corpse for a minimum of 1 minute. So a 25-minute practice, for example, needs a minimum 5-minute Corpse.

By the same token, you shouldn't be a slave to your watch. If something is hurting or tingling in a pose before the allotted time is up, then by all means come out. Use your watch wisely.

Traditional Benefit

Pond Seal is an excellent way to open an asana or *pranayama* practice. It's also a useful preliminary exercise for the Flying-Up Bond (*uddiyana bandha*). Gheranda claims that Pond prevents you from growing old (*jara*) and dying, which is probably enough incentive to give it serious consideration.

Caution

If your fingers start to tingle when doing this exercise, immediately raise the backs of your hands with a thickly folded blanket underneath the hands, with the sandbag on top of the hands. If the tingling persists, remove the bag and widen your arms beyond than shoulder-width.

Variation

After you've stretched your arms back, but before you've straightened your legs, stack your left knee on top of your right. Exhale and slowly lower your legs to the left, onto the inner edge of your right foot. Be sure not to force the legs to the floor; take them over just until you feel an easy stretch along the right side of your torso, keeping your right shoulder blade on the floor. Use the top knee to press *out*, not down, on the bottom knee, so that it seems to lengthen away from the pelvis. As you do this, reach actively in the opposite direction through the right arm. Direct your inhalations into the right ribs, expanding with each intake and releasing the belly with each exhalation. Hold for 1 to 2 minutes, inhale up, unstack your knees and repeat the pose to the right for the same length of time. Come up with another inhalation.

BIRD CATCHER SEAL (PASHINI MUDRA)

PASHIN · bird catcher (from *pasha*, meaning a snare, bond, chain; especially the noose as an attribute of Shiva or Yama, the personification of death)

Nowadays this position is called Yoga Sleep Pose (*yoga nidrasana*, see *Light on Yoga* #146), but it's easy to see why it might be called the Bird Catcher too—the practitioner's body seems like a bird snared in a net (*pasha*). Is there a hidden meaning here too? Perhaps the "bird" is the breath, which is often compared to a wild goose or swan, because it's a vehicle that will lift us to "heaven," that is, higher consciousness. Is the breath somehow "caught" in this seal, allowing us to use it for transformative purposes?

LITTLE LAMP: YOGA SLEEP
(YOGA NIDRA)

The story goes that the yogi makes his bed in the Yoga Sleep Pose; his "legs form . . . the pillow and the back is his couch."[1] The reference to "sleep" here has a deeper meaning. We all know or experience two basic states of consciousness, waking and sleep (we'll say dreaming is a substate of sleep). But the yogis say that what we think of as "waking" is actually a kind of sleep called *avidya* ("not knowing"), so even though we're walking around with our eyes wide open, we're actually spiritually asleep to our authentic identity. For the yogis, though, the situation is exactly reversed: while asleep to the distracting allure of the world and

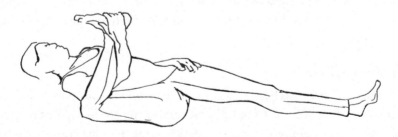

Fig. 2. Bird Catcher Seal (*pashini mudra*).

the limitations of ego identity, they're wide awake to their true self. So yoga sleep is a kind of paradox: defined in spiritual terms, the sleeper is, in fact, fully awake spiritually.

Now if you looked at the full pose, you might be thinking, "He stored Rooster because he thinks it's too difficult and substituted *this* pose instead?" I'm not suggesting that we perform the full Bird Catcher; rather, we'll do a modification that follows well from Pond Seal and serves as a general warm-up for the groins.

Practice

On an exhalation, lift your bent right thigh to your belly, keeping your left foot on the floor. Bring your right arm against the *inside* of your right leg and press your elbow against the back of your thigh just above the knee. Cross the arm to the outside of the ankle and grip the *outside* of the foot. Draw your right thigh in close to the right side of your torso and raise your right foreleg perpendicular to the floor. Snuggle the back of your right shoulder against your inner right knee as closely as possible, and firmly press your right thigh toward the floor.

Are you a bit tight in the groins? You'll know the answer fairly quickly in this pose. If you are, keep the left knee bent with the foot on the floor. You might also feel the base of your skull being pulled down onto the back of your neck, so you might need to rest your head on a thickly folded blanket. But if you have some room in the groins, then you can extend the left leg as you did for Pond Seal. Press out strongly through the left heel and make the thigh heavy on the floor.

Hold this pose anywhere from 1 to 3 minutes, then repeat on the left side for the same length of time. Finally, roll yourself up into the Wind-Freeing Pose for a minute or so, before moving on to the next step in the sequence.

Traditional Benefit

Traditional Bird Catcher is said to awaken *shakti,* another name for *kundalini.* Since this isn't the full pose, and we're not in the business of stirring up any slumbering serpents, let's just say that this exercise opens the groins.

SECTION 2: LOTUS WARM-UP (1)

There are five poses in this section, and all but one (Lion Pose) are found only in the *Gheranda-Samhita*. These poses form a logical sequence that prepares the thighs, groins, and ankles for Lotus Pose (in Section 4).

General caution: All five poses are kneeling poses, which means you need to be extra careful with the knees. If you're unable to sit comfortably in any of these poses, be sure to sit on a high support, such as a foam block or thickly folded blanket.

LITTLE LAMP: SITTING SUPPORT

About half of the thirty-two asanas in the Original sequence are floor-sitting poses. This can be a problem for us Westerners because most of us are primarily chair-sitters, which isn't conducive to floor-sitting. When we get down and sit on the floor, we often have a difficult time bringing our pelvis into a neutral position. We tend to slump on the back of the sitting bones, so our tailbone is much closer to the floor than the pubic bone, which results in a flattened or outwardly rounded lower back. Even when the torso is in the upright position, this back-tilted pelvis puts a strain on the lower back and neck, and then if we bend forward or twist, an already bad situation is exacerbated.

How do you know if you need a blanket or not? Take my word for it, you probably do; but if you don't believe me, try this simple test. Sit flat on the floor with your legs extended out in front of your torso. Rest your hands on your hips, fingers in front near the hip points, thumbs behind on the top rim of the pelvis near the base of the sacrum (which is actually the base of the spine). Judge honestly now, which are higher, the fingers or the thumbs? For most people, I'd be willing to bet cash money that it's the former and that the latter are much closer to the floor. In other words, it's that back-tilted pelvis I was just talking about, and with any forward bend or twist (and most likely even a backbend), it's a strained lower back waiting to happen. I'm not trying to scare you, only convince you that if you're not accustomed to using a blanket support when sitting on the floor, now might be a good time to start.

The next obvious question is, if I'm supposed to use a lift, how do I know how high the lift should be? The obvious answer is high enough to bring your pelvis at least to neutral, so the pubic bone and tailbone are equidistant from the floor. For some of us, that means just an inch or two; for others, it might mean sitting on a thick bolster. Don't skimp on the height; it's better to sit too high than too low.

Try this. Fold one of your yoga blankets into a square or rectangle about 2 or 3 inches thick. Sit on one of the firm or folded edges of the blanket, legs stretched out on the floor in what we call Staff Pose (*dandasana*; see *Light on Yoga* #34). Since the sitting bones are shaped like a pair of rocking-chair rockers on the bottom of your pelvis, rock back and forth slowly for a minute or so. Start out with exaggerated movements, getting a sense of the two extremes of the rocking movement. Slow down gradually until you come to a stop more or less at the midpoint of the two extremes, on the "bottom" (or slightly forward of the bottom) of the rocker. Make your thigh bones very heavy, and firm your shoulder blades and sacrum against your back torso.

Now bring your hands on the top rim of your pelvis again. Where are the fingers and thumbs relative to the floor now? Is the rim more or less parallel, or does it seem that the back pelvis is still drooping down? If your answer is yes to the first part of this question, then you have the proper height; if yes applies to the second part, then you need to sit slightly higher. Keep adding to your support's height an inch at a time until you can safely say that your pelvis is in a relatively neutral position. Stay in this pose for 1 to 2 minutes.

DIAMOND POSE (VAJRASANA)

> *VAJRA* · diamond, adamantine; hard, impenetrable; thunderbolt (from *vaj*, "to be hard or strong")

Diamond is a simple sitting-on-the-heels position, just a step away from the modern version of Hero Pose (see Section 4), in which the buttocks are settled between the heels, either on the floor or on a support. I say "modern version" here because traditional Hero (at least as it's explained in the *Gheranda-Samhita*) is slightly different, and we'll come to the traditional version in Section 4. Although I'm translating *vajra* into English as Diamond, it can also be rendered as Thunderbolt. I chose the former because three of my sources agree that, according to Gheranda's instruction, we're to sit in this pose with our thighs (*jangha*) as "hard" or "tight" as diamonds.

LITTLE LAMP: WHAT IS *JANGHA*?

Now I don't want to be too literal about this, and I'm not faulting Gheranda's anatomical training, but taken at face value, making your thighs "tight" in this pose doesn't seem right. If we want to sit on our heels in Diamond, the thigh muscles (or quadriceps, which when contracted straighten or extend the knee) have to release. If they're tight, we won't be able to bend or flex our knees and get our buttocks down on our heels. To confuse the issue further, a fourth source has Gheranda telling us to make the "lower legs" (presumably the shins and/or calves) hard. Once again, this doesn't make anatomical sense. To sit in Diamond, our front ankles must also release so the tops of our feet can rest comfortably on the floor. If the shin muscles are tight, that can't happen — or at least, it can't happen easily. So what gives?

It turns out that the word *jangha* in the original instruction can be interpreted in three ways: as "shin" or "shank"; as the "upper part of the leg . . . about the loins," which seems to indicate the thigh; and as "leg" in general. The question then is, which half of the leg is Gheranda referring to, upper or lower, or is he referring to the whole limb? The answer

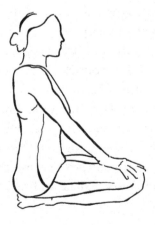

Fig. 3. Diamond Pose (*vajrasana*).

is, of course, we'll never know. I can't say how each of my sources would justify his definition, but I'm sure they're all perfectly reasonable. For practicality's sake though, I'll go out on a limb—a lower limb specifically—and interpret *jangha* as "leg." If Gheranda knew anything about anatomy, he wouldn't advise us to make any of the muscles along the front leg hard in this pose. I propose that Gheranda wasn't making reference to leg *muscles* at all, but to the way the legs should be arranged in the pose. That is to say, he wants us—or maybe I just want him to want us—to bring the legs "adamantly" together in two ways: first, to flex the knees completely so that the back thighs press firmly against the calves, and second, to press the inner legs together just as firmly. This makes the legs figuratively impenetrable; nothing can get through from the sides (between the thighs and calves) or the front (between the inner thighs).

Practice

To begin Diamond, rest on the floor on all fours, with your knees directly below your hips and your hands directly below your shoulders. You might take this opportunity to rock the pelvis to and fro a few times, pressing the tailbone toward the floor so you flex (round) the spine (on an exhalation), and lifting the sitting bones toward the ceiling so you extend (arch) the spine (on an inhalation) a few times. This is commonly called Cat-Cow Pose, presumably the former is the rounded-spine position, and the latter is the arched-spine position. I personally don't favor this terminology, preferring the more down-to-earth, less imaginative, All-Fours Pose. Whatever you call it, work the movements slowly, distributing the movements evenly throughout the entire length of the spine.

Now press your inner thighs, knees, calves, and feet together, and spread the tops of your feet on the floor. Lift your hands off the floor, bring your thighs and torso upright (perpendicular to the floor), and press your palms together in *anjali mudra*. Hold for 30 seconds to 1 minute, perhaps taking the time to dedicate yourself to the practice at hand and your practice, in turn, to the service of the self—though it's up to you to determine how best to begin your practice, even to just moving directly into the pose from All-Fours. Exhale and sit back on your heels.

LITTLE LAMP: ANJALI MUDRA

ANJALI • the open hands placed side by side and slightly
hollowed (as if by a beggar to receive food; when raised to
the forehead, a mark of supplication); reverence, salutation, benediction

The well-known *anjali mudra* is performed today with the hands pressed
firmly together, but as you can see from the preceding definition, it's
technically a cupped-hands gesture of supplication. Energetically, it
symbolizes the joining of the two complementary energies of the body-
mind—the solar *ha* (right hand) and the lunar *tha* (left hand). Practi-
cally speaking, by spreading the palms evenly against each other, you can
create a similar spreading of the shoulder blades against the back. For
more on hand seals (*hasta mudras*), see chapter 6.

Sitting

There are two different ways to sit in this pose, depending on how we
interpret the instruction to "place the feet on either side of the anus"
(*guda*). One version takes what we might call a "narrow" approach, so
that the buttocks are resting right on the heels. The second version takes
a "broad" approach, so that the buttocks are snuggled down between
the heels and sit, as if in a saddle, on the inner arches. Because the first
version bears the weight of the body directly down on the heels, it seems
to stretch the front of the ankles a bit more, while the second version
seems slightly easier on the ankles. You can decide for yourself which
way to play this one. But if your knees protest, wedge a thickly folded
blanket between the backs of your thighs and your calves; if it's your
ankles protesting, roll up a towel and put it between your ankles and
the floor.

Hands

Gheranda doesn't say what to do with your hands in Diamond. The simplest course of action is to lay them on your thighs, palms down, or stack
them in your lap, with the back of one hand nesting in the palm of the

other. You might cup your hands over your knees, or press your palms against your soles, with the bases of the palms on the heels, fingers pointing to the toes. You might also fold your forearms across your chest and hold the opposite elbow with each hand, or cross your forearms in front of your torso and slip each hand into the opposite armpit.

Stay in this pose anywhere from 1 to 3 minutes. During this time, perform Skull Brightening. When you're ready to come out, exhale and lean forward onto your hands again in All-Fours. In this position, you're ready for the next pose.

Traditional Benefit

Gheranda claims that Diamond brings the yogi *siddhi*. This word crops up again and again in the *Gheranda-Samhita* and *Hatha-Yoga-Pradipika,* and it's hard to say exactly what it means—a lot depends on its context. Three of my five translators agree on "success" as the proper rendering; the other two chime in with "perfection" and "psychic powers." We'll go into this fascinating word when we come to its namesake asana, *siddhasana.* For now, let's just go with the majority opinion and interpret *siddha* as "success," although we're not either on what kind of success we can expect.

Variation

From Diamond, inhale, lean your torso back and press your palms against the floor, just behind your feet, fingers pointing forward toward your feet. Straighten your elbows, press your shoulder blades firmly against your back torso, and lift the top of your sternum toward the ceiling. This will stretch the front of your torso and shoulders. Hold for a minute or so, then come up with an inhalation, leading with your chest, your head trailing.

To increase this stretch while your hands are on the floor, inhale and lift your buttocks off your heels or inner feet. Lengthen your tailbone toward the backs of your knees, and stretch the front of your body from your knees to your shoulders.

Instead of placing the tops of your feet on the floor when you sit on your heels, turn your toes under so the balls of your feet are on the floor and your heels are elevated. You can sit back on your heels or, if that's too painful, on a yoga block set between your feet. You can cup your hands on your knees or press your palms together in *anjali mudra*. This is a good preparation for traditional Superior Pose (see Section 7).

With your toes turned under, you can spread your knees wide apart. From here, you can lean your torso forward, rest your hands on the floor and your head on your knees, and salute your guru or teacher. It's also possible to recline the torso in Diamond, though with the tops of the feet on the floor and the toes not turned under. Beginning students are likely to need some support under the back of the torso, either one or more thickly folded blankets or a yoga bolster.

LITTLE LAMP: *VAJRA*

Once upon a time, the gods and demons had a war (yet another one) and, assisted by the scary Vritra (whose name means "Encloser" because he covered the world in darkness), the demons won. As usual, the gods ran off to Grandfather Brahma for help, who advised them, "If you want to defeat the demons, you must kill Vritra." Kill Vritra? How? Vritra wasn't your run-of-the mill demon; according to one account, he looked like a volcano, with burning eyes, a huge mouth that "drank up the sky," and terrible fangs.

The gods decided they needed a special weapon against such a formidable foe. So they went to an ascetic named Dadhichi who had diamond-hard thunderbolts for bones. The gods asked Dadhichi to donate his bones to their cause, and Dadhichi, who was devoted to helping others, agreed. He immediately surrendered his body and ascended to heaven in a rain of flowers. The divine artisan Vishvakarman ("All Doer," also known as Tvashtri, or "Carpenter") fashioned Dadhichi's bones ("Dadhichi's bones," or *dadhica ashti*, is another name for the thunderbolt) into a mighty thunderbolt (*vajra*, the "hard or mighty one"); in some accounts it was shaped like a discus and in others like a pair of bolts crossed like an X. It was taken as a weapon by the Indian sky god Indra, the rough equivalent of the Greek's chief god, Zeus.

In the great battle that ensued, Vritra seemed to get the better of the gods' leader and clean-up hitter Indra, swallowing the poor fellow whole. But Indra was no slouch: using his thunderbolt, he sliced his way out of

Vritra's belly and cut off the demon's head. In the end, the gods defeated the demons.

The thunderbolt is always the weapon of choice of the most powerful sky gods—not only Indra, but also the Greek Zeus and the Norse Thor. It represents both destruction and justice—just ask Vritra—as well as creation (*vajra* is a secret name for "penis"). The *vajra* is also a diamond and, as the hardest substance, can cut through all other substances. In the spiritual realm, the diamond stands for authentic self-knowledge that can cut through and free us from the fetter of self-ignorance (*avidya*).

Lion Pose (Simhasana)

SIMHA · lion, powerful one, hero, eminent person

Lion Pose is described in both the *Hatha-Yoga-Pradipika* and the *Gheranda-Samhita*. Svatmarama gives a slightly more detailed account and includes Lion among the four best asanas of the fifteen he lists. He praises the pose by saying it's honored, even worshipped (*pujita*) by the "best yogis" (*yogi pungava*).

But neither Svatmarama nor Gheranda mentions two of the most characteristic elements of the modern version of Lion—its curled-out tongue and its roaring lionlike exhalation through a wide-open mouth.

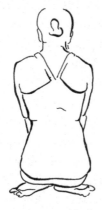 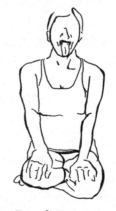

Fig. 4a. Lion Pose (*simhasana*), back.

Fig. 4b. Lion Pose (*simhasana*), front.

One possible answer is supplied by *Asana Pranayama Mudra Bandha*. The traditional pose represents a condition of alert readiness often seen in cats, in which the "lion is sitting quietly, waiting for something to happen. This is the mental attitude the mind has to adopt in order to enter deep meditative states."[2] This pose includes the roar one book calls *simha garjana*, literally the "roaring lion," which is, to mix metaphors, a horse of a different color.

Practice

From Diamond, lift your buttocks off your heels and lean onto your hands in All-Fours. Cross your right ankle under the left, then sit back and snuggle your perineum down onto your top (left) heel. One of my translations says to put the shins on the floor (actually, Gheranda uses the word *bhumi*, or "ground," presumably because his audience was practicing outdoors); another recommends the "front part of the head of the tibia," which seems more accurate. (Note, however, the Iyengar version in *Light on Yoga* #49, in which the knee of the top ankle is off the floor.) Press your palms against the same-side knees and spread your fingers wide (according to Svatmarama) like a lion's exposed claws. Open your mouth wide (neither Svatmarama nor Gheranda say anything about stretching out the tongue as we do nowadays) and apply Net-Bearing Bond (mentioned only by Gheranda). You can use the pressure of the hands against the knees to help firm the shoulder blades against the back and lift the chest, an action essential to avoid straining the back of the neck during Net-Bearing. With your eyes open wide, stare at the tip of your nose (*nasa agra*) with an "intently absorbed mind" (*susamahita*).

GARJANA

> *GARJANA* · crying, roaring, rumbling (of clouds), growl, grunt; passion; battle; excessive indignation, reproach

Here is where both versions end, as I noted earlier, without mention of the famous Lion exhalation. Stretch the tongue out of the mouth, curl the tip down toward the chin, and supply the *garjana* yourself three times with the ankles crossed left over right. Now lean forward on your hands in All-Fours and reverse the ankle cross, left under right; sit back and repeat the Lion's roar three more times. Between each exhalation, lift your head out of Net-Bearing and take a few normal breaths. Finally, lean forward to All-Fours again, uncross your ankles, touch your inner big toes together, and get ready for the next pose.

LITTLE LAMP: MODERN GARJANA (HISSING)

The Lion's roar is similar to a modern technique developed by our friend Mabel Elsworth Todd. In her book, *The Thinking Body,* she describes hissing as a way to release tension and improve breathing. Lie supine on the floor, knees bent, feet on the floor, arms crossed over your front torso in what's called the Constructive Rest Position. Hiss out through your partially closed teeth several times, making sure not to gasp between hisses. According to Todd, "The spine will lengthen, the body become more narrow and the pressure on the vertebrae more even upon the floor." She concludes that this balance relaxes the body and is the "great conservator of energy."[3] Hissing is an excellent prelude to asana practice, Corpse Pose, or *pranayama.*

Traditional Benefit

Svatmarama says that Lion "facilitates the three *bandhas*" (*Hatha-Yoga-Pradipika* 1.52), by which he means the three major bonds: Net-Bearing (by strengthening the throat muscles); Root (by contracting the perineum as you sit on the upper heel); and Flying-Up (by contracting the belly muscle to power the Lion exhalation). Gheranda claims that Lion destroys all disease (*vyadhi*). *Hatha-Tatva-Kaumudi* 7.16 notes that through this pose, the subtle energy channels (*nadis*) regain normal functioning—a must as a preliminary for *pranayama*—and the hands (*hastas*) and feet (*padas*) gain lightness (*laghava*).

Caution

If you're not accustomed to performing Net-Bearing Bond, be sure to spend some time practicing this technique before applying it to Lion Pose.

For various reasons, some students find the leg position in this pose impossibly painful. If the pressure of the top ankle on the bottom is too extreme, try putting a rolled-up towel between them for padding. If this doesn't help, or if you have pain in one or both of your knees, simply sit on the floor with your shins crossed in front of your torso.

Variation

In one variation of Lion, you turn your toes under and sit on your raised heels with your knees spread wide. Press your palms to the floor between your legs, tips of the thumbs touching. Open your mouth wide, stretch out your tongue, and gaze at the tip of your nose. Again, the instructions say nothing about the Lion exhalation, which you may supply yourself. You may also use the crossed-ankle position of Lion as simple sitting pose, laying your hands lightly on your knees and directing your gaze between your eyebrows.

LITTLE LAMP: *VYAGHRA*

Another traditional name for this pose is *vyaghrasana,* or Tiger Pose (*vyaghra,* for "tiger; any preeminently strong or noble person"). I know what you're thinking: this word sounds familiar. The Sanskrit *vyaghra* sounds very much like a well-known drug that treats a certain "dysfunction." There seem to be a few doubters out there who think the similarity between the two words is a coincidence, but most commentators agree that the drug name is taken from the Sanskrit.

FROG POSE (MANDUKASANA)

MANDUKA · frog

Frog might be considered a variation of Diamond, the difference being the width of the knees and, depending on how you sit in Diamond, the placement of the buttocks on the feet.

Practice

From Lion Pose, lean forward, uncross your ankles, and bring your feet side by side as they were for Diamond. Touch your inner big toes together, but keep your heels apart. Exhale and sit back in the "saddle" of your inner feet, so that your buttocks nestle down between your heels and rest on the curves of your inner arches. Slide your knees apart as far as you comfortably can, at least to the width of your sticky mat but wider if possible.

Hands

Gheranda doesn't say what to do with your hands in Frog. The simplest thing is to cup each around the same-side knee or just lay them, palms down, on the thighs. The *Hatha-Ratna-Avali* (3.55) suggests slipping the hands underneath and gripping the shins, and another text says to cross the wrists and press the hands lightly against the chest. Stay in this position anywhere from 1 to 3 minutes.

Traditional Benefit

None listed.

Caution

The cautions noted for Diamond also apply to Frog.

Variation

As you did for the Diamond variation, turn your toes under so that the balls of your feet are on the floor and your heels are elevated. Then sit on your heels with wide knees.

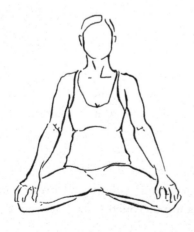

Fig. 5. Frog Pose (*mandukasana*).

LITTLE LAMP: *MANDUKA*

If you want to say "frog" in English, you're pretty much stuck with that word, though I suppose a lot of people will know what you're talking about if you use "croaker." But Sanskrit has at least a dozen words for "frog" besides *manduka*. Among the host of frogs is *ajambha* ("toothless") and *ajihva* ("tongueless"); *bhakabhakaya; bheka* (which is probably a word that imitates the croaking of frogs); *dardura* ("frog's bite"); *jihmamohana* (*jihma*, "crooked, dishonest, to miss one's aim," and *mohana*, "bewildered"); *katurava* ("frog"); *luluka* ("frog"); *plavaga* (literally "going by leaps"); *varshabhu* (literally "produced in the rains"), and *varshagosha* ("uttering cries in the rainy season," meaning a large frog, from *varsha*, "raining").

I suppose it's no surprise that there's a mantra in praise of frogs in the *Rigveda*, Hinduism's holiest book. It playfully compares the croaking of frogs revived at the start of the rainy season to the chants of Brahmin priests at a sacrifice (*Rigveda* 7.103:2, 7; translation by Wendy Doniger O'Flaherty):

> When the heavenly waters came upon him dried out like a leather bag, lying in the pool, then the cries of the frogs joined in chorus like the lowing of cows with calves . . .
>
> Like Brahmins at the over-night sacrifice . . . so you frogs around a pool celebrate the day of the year when the rains come.

RAISED FROG POSE (UTTANA MANDUKASANA)

UTTANA · raised, upright

Raised Frog is a continuation of Frog. The legs and torso remain in the same position, but the arms are raised to form what's called Most Excellent Seal (*jyeshtha mudra*), which aims to stretch the upper torso and armpits.

Preliminary
In Frog, inhale and raise your right arm straight toward the ceiling. Bend the elbow and touch the palm to your upper right back, just above the

shoulder blade. Keep the inner right arm close to the side of your head. Now reach your left hand over your crown and grip your right elbow. Pull the right elbow up toward the ceiling and slightly back, stretching the back of the upper right arm and armpit. Hold for 30 seconds to 1 minute. Release the elbow and reverse arms, repeating for the same length of time on the left.

Practice

Now inhale and raise both arms straight toward the ceiling. Rotate the arms so the palms face the wall behind you, then exhale, bend both elbows and rest the palms on the upper back, near the same-side shoulder blades. Lift the elbows toward the ceiling and lightly squeeze the sides of your head with the inner arms. Hold this position for 1 minute, then release the arms.

There are three versions of the next pose, Tortoise, coming up. If you're doing Tortoise 1 (for beginners), stay in Frog. For Tortoise 2 (for intermediates) and 3 (the full pose), bring your feet on the floor in front of your torso.

Traditional Benefit
None listed.

Caution
The cautions noted for Diamond also apply to Raised Frog.

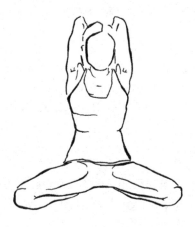

Fig. 6. Raised Frog Pose (*uttana mandukasana*).

Variation

Instead of touching the palms to the same-side shoulder blades, cross the wrists and touch the palms to the opposite-side shoulder blades. Hold the first cross for the first half of your stay in the pose, then reverse the cross for the second half.

Another way to arrange your arms is to cross your forearms above your head, and hold the elbows with the opposite-side hands. As in the preceding variation, hold the first cross for the first half of your stay in the pose, then reverse for the second half.

Tortoise Pose (Kurmasana)

KURMA · tortoise, turtle

You might be familiar with the modern version of Tortoise (see *Light on Yoga* #133) that, with its humped back and protruding arms and legs, is indeed reminiscent of a tortoise. This pose isn't, however, easily accessible to most students. Nor is Gheranda's traditional version easily performed by the average student (for a different reason), but to visualize it as a tortoise requires a stretch of the imagination. Gheranda's Tortoise is similar to Diamond, save in one respect: the feet are rotated or turned outward (*vyutkrama*, "inverted order, out of the right course") so the inner edges are pressed on the floor with the toes pointing off to the sides.

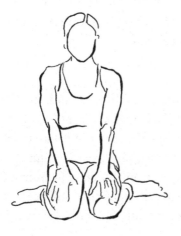

Fig. 7. Tortoise Pose (*kurmasana*).

You might already be wincing as you think about performing this difficult feat, but I'll give you three versions to work with, the first two of which will take some of the sting out of the full pose.

Practice 1: For Beginners

Release your arms from Raised Frog and hook your thumbs under the flaps of muscle at the front of your armpits (the pectoralis major). Lift and pull up on the muscle, spread the other fingers across the front of your chest and rest them to either side of the sternum. Exhale, lean forward, and rest your elbows and forehead or chin on the floor, with your elbows pointing out to the sides and your forearms pressed against the fronts of your knees.

To me, this position looks a lot more like a tortoise than the pose described in Gheranda. It's similar to what we call Child's Pose (*balasana*), except instead of laying the arms on the floor, palms up, beside the hips, the thumbs are hooked in the front armpits. Students commonly take Child's Pose as a resting position, which it is, but too often they forget that resting isn't the same as spacing out. As with Child's Pose, this version of Tortoise, with the front torso pressed against the inner thighs, provides an excellent opportunity to practice breathing into the back torso and lungs. It may sound strange, but most of us breathe primarily in the front torso and lungs, leaving the back mostly "unbreathed."

So remember to direct your inhalations into the space between the shoulder blades, and use the breath to create space across the back torso from side to side. On each exhalation, soften your groins and allow your torso to rest more completely on your inner thighs. Stay in this pose for 1 to 3 minutes, then come up with an inhalation.

Practice 2: For Intermediates

This is a variation of the full pose as described by Gheranda and might be called either Half-Tortoise Pose (*ardha kurmasana*) or One-Foot Tortoise Pose (*eka pada kurmasana*). You may be able to sit flat on the floor, but it's more likely you'll need some support, such as a block, under your buttocks. Start with your knees bent, feet on the floor in front of the torso. Lean slightly to your left, and with the right knee still bent, swing your right foot to the outside of your right hip. Press the *inner* foot and knee to the floor so that the back heel is beside the hip and the toes point away to the right. If you've not already done so, you might need to pad the floor underneath the inside of the foot and knee. Now *carefully* lower the right buttock back to the floor or support. Be sure that both sitting bones rest comfortably on something, either the floor or a block, and that the inner knee isn't strained. If you can't rest back to the right easily, or if you feel strain in the knee, then raise yourself off the floor or onto a higher block support.

But if this is fairly easy for you, then lower your support (if you're sitting on one) or sit on the floor. If it's still easy with the heel beside the hip, good for you. Slide the foot farther away from the hip until you feel the right buttock start to lift or the right shin is parallel to the front edge of the sticky mat. Stay for 1 to 3 minutes, then lean back to the left, use your right hand to lift your right knee off the floor, and stand your right foot back on the floor. Repeat with the left leg for the same length of time.

Variation

Bring the right foot into Half-Tortoise and the left heel into the perineum (like Perfected Pose, see Section 11). After a minute or two, reverse the feet.

Practice 3: Full Tortoise

Let's break the full version down into variations A and B. For Tortoise 3A, sit either flat on the floor or on a block support (it might be necessary to use more than one block to create sufficient height), with your knees bent and your feet on the floor in front of the torso. Lean slightly forward; swing one heel and then the other to the outside of its same-side hip, resting the inner feet and knees on the floor, toes pointing away from the torso. Sit back on the floor or your support.

In the traditional pose, which we'll call Tortoise 3B, sit on the outer heels with the inner feet and knees resting on the floor. As I mentioned earlier, this can be considered a challenging variation of Diamond.

Hands

The simplest hand position is to lay each on the same-side knee, palms down. Alternatively, as described in the mild Tortoise version, you can hook your thumbs in their same-side armpits, with your fingers spread across your chest.

Stay for 1 to 3 minutes, then lean forward. Remove one leg, *keeping the knee completely flexed,* and stand the foot on the floor. Drop the entire outer leg to the side on the floor so the hip joint is rotated outward (laterally), straighten the leg off to the side, and then swing it back to center in front of the torso from the hip. Bounce the knee gently on the floor a few times. Repeat with the other leg.

Traditional Benefit
None listed.

LITTLE LAMP: *KURMA*

I imagine most of us are familiar with Aesop's fable of the Tortoise and the Hare, how the former plugs along and wins the race against all odds — with an assist from the latter's arrogance and inattention, two qualities that mark the Hare as a nonyogi. In India, the tortoise plays a significant role in several well-known stories. In a Vedic creation story, his lower shell becomes the earth and his upper shell the sky. In the story of the Churning of the Ocean, he's an avatar of the deity Vishnu and, diving deep into the ocean, serves as the base for the mountain-sized churning stick. And in the *Bhagavad-Gita* (2.56), his ability to draw his head and limbs into his shell to protect himself from the slings and arrows of the outside world is compared to a yogi drawing his usually outgoing senses into the protective shell of his own consciousness — a practice known as *pratyahara,* literally "drawing back, withdrawal"—in preparation for meditation. According to Krishna (translation by Graham Schweig), when successful, the yogi is "undisturbed in suffering ... free from desire in all kinds of happiness, whose passion, fear, and anger have departed. ..."

Caution
I'll emphasize again the importance of protecting your knees in the medium and intense versions. Be aware of what your knee feels like, not only in the pose, but also for the next few days after practicing it. If any

strain shows up, be sure to change the way you practice Tortoise, either moving back down the ladder to the previous variation or raising your buttocks off (or higher off) the floor.

LITTLE LAMP: GARUDA

GARUDA · devourer

If asked to define *garuda,* most students would hazard "eagle." This isn't exactly wrong—Garuda is the *name* of an eagle, or at least an eaglelike creature, the king of the birds, who's also the special mount of Vishnu—but literally the word means "devourer." This seems like a strange name for an eagle, until we learn the story of his birth: he was so bright he frightened the gods, who identified him with the devouring fire of the sun's rays. (However, Alain Danielou derives *garuda* from *gri,* "to speak," and translates the word as "wings of speech," since here he represents the words of the Vedas, which can transport humans to the heavenly world.)

Nowadays *garudasana* is a pretzel-like standing pose (see *Light on Yoga* #23) popularly called Eagle. As you can see from the preceding story, though it was the name of an eagle, *garuda* itself means "devourer." In the *Gheranda-Samhita,* this pose is a sitting position similar to Tortoise. This pose is optional.

Practice

From Tortoise, slip your feet from under your buttocks out to the sides of your hips. Rest your hands on your knees.

Traditional Benefit

None listed.

SECTION 3: LOTUS WARM-UP (2)

There are two more Lotus preparations in this section that continue our work with the thighs, groins, and ankles.

FORTUNATE POSE (BHADRASANA)

BHADRA • blessed, auspicious, fortunate, prosperous,
happy, good, gracious, friendly, kind, excellent, beautiful

We might call Gheranda's version of Fortunate Pose "reversed" Tortoise
(see Section 2), because the ankles and feet are reversed. But instead of the
feet resting on their inner arches with the toes pointing out to the sides,
they rest on the inner arches with the toes pointing *straight back* and the
knees spread wide as in Frog. Nowadays this pose is called the Bound Root
Pose (*mula bandhasana;* see *Light on Yoga* #165). This foot position isn't
accessible to the average student—or even the above-average student—
so for the traditional sequence, we'll use a variation of Svatmarama's version of Fortunate, which we call Bound Angle Pose (*baddha konasana*). In
Svatmarama's version, the ankles are set below the perineum (*sivan*), but
we'll just draw the heels up comfortably to the pubic bone.

Practice

Sit on your support, lean back slightly, and bring your soles together, releasing your knees downward. Draw your heels as close to your perineum
as you comfortably can. Now this is important: press the soles firmly together and push the knees *away* from the pelvis, as if widening them out
to the sides, but *not* down toward the floor.

If you're stiffer in the groins, reach down and hold on to your ankles,
or just lay your palms on your knees in Yogini Pose (*yogini,* "female practitioner or goddess"). More flexible students can lace their fingers and

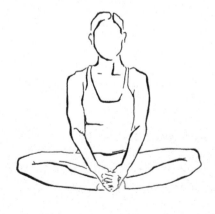

Fig. 8. Fortunate Pose
(*bhadrasana*).

wrap their hands around the top four pairs of toes. Leave the little toes out of the grip, and press them firmly into the floor. Use the pull of the hands on the feet or ankles to help press the shoulder blades against the back torso and lift the chest.

Now lean the torso forward to increase the stretch in the groins, but as usual, come down only from the groins and not the belly. Imagine the sacrum pressing deep into the back of your pelvis and, still lifting the top of the sternum, exhale slightly forward. Stay in this pose anywhere from 1 to 5 minutes.

Traditional Benefit

Both Svatmarama and Gheranda agree that Fortunate "destroys" (*vin-asha*) disease.

Caution

If you have a serious groin or knee injury, only perform Fortunate with a blanket supporting each of the outer thighs. Raise the knees slightly *higher* than the fullest stretch of your inner groins. Remember: never force your knees down toward the floor; instead, release the heads of the thighbones. When this action leads, the knees follow.

Little Lamp: Cobbler's Pose

Svatmarama notes that "accomplished" or "perfected" yogins call this Goraksha's Pose. Fortunate Pose is also known informally as Cobbler's Pose. As Iyengar notes, "This is how Indian cobblers sit."[4]

Bull Pose (Vrishasana)

VRISHA · male of any species, bull, strong or potent man; the chief among members, such as the thumb; a piece of ground suitable for the foundation of a house

It would be fitting if Bull had some kind of relationship to Cow Face, but the two don't have much in common. We can think of Bull as a "half-and-half" pose, half-Frog and half-Fortunate.

Practice

From Fortunate, lean to the left and grasp your right ankle. Pick your foot up and, keeping your knee completely flexed, swivel it around to the outside of your right hip. As you do, slide your right knee off to the side, so that your right leg is in a Frog-like position. Rest the top of your foot on the floor with the toes pointing straight back, leaving a thumb's-width space between the outer hip and the inner heel. If you want to be technically correct, you can set your right heel under your anus (*payu mula*). Tuck the left heel comfortably up near the pubic bone.

You may find that you're tilting over somewhat (or more than somewhat) toward the Fortunate leg, which may or may not be a problem for you. The tight hip muscles that are creating the tilt will eventually release, the raised buttock will sit on the floor, and all will be well. As a temporary measure, slip a folded blanket under the hip of the Fortunate leg, making it high enough to help the torso tilt back to neutral.

Stay in this position for 1 to 3 minutes. Then lean to the left, grab the right ankle again, and — still keeping the knee completely flexed — swivel the foot back to Fortunate. Lean to the right and repeat with the left leg, staying in the pose for the same length of time as you did on the first side. Then lean back to the right and bring the left leg back to Fortunate.

Traditional Benefit

None listed.

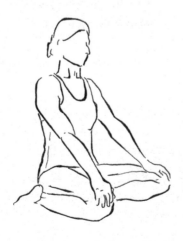

Fig. 9. Bull Pose (*vrishasana*).

LITTLE LAMP: FEMALE YOGIS

Bull and Cow (Face) are the only two "mated" poses in the *Gheranda-Samhita*, unless you count the spiritual mating of Matsyendra and his supposed pupil, Goraksha. Cow is the only obviously "female" pose in the lineup, which suggests an interesting question: were there any female yogis (*yogini*) in Gheranda's time, or is female participation in yoga a modern phenomenon? According to David Gordon White, there were indeed cults of yoginis as far back as at least the sixth century C.E., though he speculates that their origins may be traced back from there many hundreds of years.[5]

But the dominance of women in yoga classes is certainly a development of the twentieth century. I've mentioned a few male pioneers of modern yoga, but who were their female counterparts? Credit should first be given to Sita Devi Yogendra, wife of Shri Yogendra, who in 1934 published *Yoga Physical Education*, the first book, as she says in her introduction, "written by a woman for women."[6]

The other early female pioneer is Eugenie Peterson, better known as Indra Devi, who first traveled to India in her late twenties, eventually became the first female student of T. Krishnamacharya, and opened a yoga school in Southern California in the late 1940s. Mataji, as she was known, wrote several popular books on yoga, including *Forever Young, Forever Healthy* (1953); *Yoga for Americans* (1959, dedicated to "my friend and pupil Gloria Swanson"); and *Renew Your Life Through Yoga* (1963).

SECTION 4: LOTUS POSES

I began the three previous sections with a brief introduction, but for this section, I'm going to be a bit more expansive. That's because I feel strongly about the safety issue with this pose, since I learned my lesson the hard way. As a young yoga student (well, young in yoga years, I was probably about thirty-five chronologically), I pursued Lotus Pose aggressively when I was totally unprepared to do so. Way back then, I decided I would watch the evening news sitting in Lotus, the first half hour with my legs crossed one way and the second half hour with them crossed the other way. This seemed to me a good way to improve my practice of this pose—and keep up on current events at the same time—and I did it most nights for several months until my inner knees began to ache and make disturbing clicking noises as I walked. I was lucky; once I stopped sitting in Lotus, the pain subsided after a few months and the clicking went away.

I sermonized at length about Lotus in the introduction to this chapter. But once again, if you're a relatively experienced student but not accustomed to performing Lotus, then I strongly urge you *not* to practice the full pose without first working with an experienced teacher. If you're a beginning student, then don't even practice Half-Lotus until getting the go-ahead from a teacher. Find someone who can accurately and fairly evaluate if your hips and groins are ready to do the pose. If you're deemed unready, then be content with either the Half-Lotus or a modified version, and depending on where you're starting, work up the ladder to the full or half version slowly. At the start of your Lotus career, don't stay in the pose for more than 5 seconds—no, that's not a misprint: *5 seconds*—and slowly add time in 5-second increments over several weeks and months. Be sure, too, if you're practicing Lotus separate from the larger sequence, to do at least a few of the preceding warm-up poses to ready your hips and groins. *Never* go into Lotus cold turkey.

Auspicious Pose (Svastikasana)

> SVASTIKA · any lucky or auspicious object (from *su,* meaning "well, good, excellent," and *asti,* meaning "being, existent." Together, these two words become *svasti,* meaning "well-being, fortune, luck, success, prosperity"; sometimes used as a term of salutation, "May it be well with you!")

Gheranda's description of Auspicious Pose is almost word for word the same as Svatmarama's. Traditionally, Auspicious is a sitting pose in what I call the Perfected Family (see Section 11), but we'll take a bit of yogic license with it and change it slightly so it serves as a preparation for Lotus Pose. This version of Auspicious is midway between Fortunate, in which the knees are spread wide, and Cow Face, in which the knees are stacked one atop the other. As you'll soon discover, it's a very effective stretch for the outer hip and buttock of the top leg.

Practice

From Fortunate, lift your knees and, keeping them bent, set your feet on the floor, heels about a foot away from your sitting bones. Slide your left heel under your right leg and set it outside your right hip, laying the outer leg on the floor. Bring your right *ankle* to the outside of your left knee. I emphasize the word *ankle* to make sure it's outside the opposite knee. Your right sole should be perpendicular to the floor, not parallel (facing up toward the ceiling). If you have difficulty getting the top leg in position, try sitting on a higher support; instead of a single folded blanket, try two, and if that still doesn't help, try sitting on a bolster.

Now lean slightly to the left and burrow the right thumb into the inner right groin. Make sure you're right in the crease between the inner thigh and pelvis. Dig the thumb deep, as if it's penetrating the skin and flesh and pushing right against the thigh bone. As with Fortunate, make sure you release the groin down, don't push the knee to the floor. Grip the outer thigh firmly and rotate it outward, that is, from the inner thigh toward the outer.

Once you've released the groin, you can keep your torso upright or lay your hands on the floor in front of your shins and lean your torso forward with an exhalation. Stay in the pose anywhere from 1 to 3 minutes. If you've leaned forward, come up on an inhalation. Return to Fortunate,

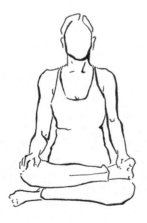

Fig. 10. Auspicious Pose (*svastikasana*).

then repeat with the left leg on top for the same length of time. Finish by returning to Fortunate.

Traditional Benefit

None listed.

Caution

I want to emphasize again that the top ankle should be outside the bottom knee and the top sole perpendicular to the floor.

Variation

Most students will get a big enough stretch in the hip of the top leg when the bottom heel is to the outside of the opposite hip. But if you find this arrangement too easy and want more of a challenge, then slide the bottom heel away from the hip and move the shin forward until you're satisfied with the stretch. Eventually the two shins will be parallel (stacked one atop the other).

LITTLE LAMP: *SVASTIKA*

A *svastika* is traditionally a good-luck or auspicious mark made on persons, places, and things. It is found in many ancient cultures from India to Egypt, from Scandinavia to South America, and all the way to Easter Island. It's shaped like a Greek cross, which has four arms of equal length, the ends of which are bent slightly to one side or the other. When bent

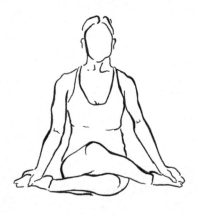

Fig. 11. Cow Face Pose (*gomukhasana*).

to the right and turning clockwise, the sign is associated with the sun and the ever-turning wheel of the universe around a fixed point. When the arms are bent left and turning counterclockwise, the mark is considered to be bad luck and inauspicious.

Cow Face Pose (Gomukhasana)

GO · cow (Sanskrit *go* is a distant relative of the English "cow")
MUKHA · face, mouth

Traditional Cow Face has the same leg position as the modern version, but neither Svatamarama nor Gheranda describe the arm position we're used to adding to this pose. Technically, the modern version should be called Bound-Hand Cow Face Pose (*baddha hasta gomukhasana*).

Little Lamp: The Cow's Face

How exactly does this pose look like a cow's face? Look at the photo in *Light on Yoga* (#37) or at yourself in a full-length mirror while in the pose. See how the legs are crossed one over the other? Those are the cow's lips. Now look at how the arms are arranged, one high and one low. Those are the cow's ears. Now do you see the face?

Practice

From Fortunate, lift your knees and, keeping them bent, set your feet on the floor, with your heels about a foot away from your sitting bones. Slide the left foot under the right knee to the outside of the right hip, laying the outer left leg on the floor. Move the left knee a little to the right until it's in line with your navel. Now stack the right knee on the left, positioning the right foot to the outside of the left hip. It's likely that the left heel will be closer to the right hip than the right heel to the left hip. If this is the case, wiggle back and forth a bit and adjust the two heels so they are as equidistant as possible from the hips. This is the traditional position for Cow Face.

Bound Hand (Baddha Hasta)

If you want to add what I assume to be the modern arm position, inhale and reach your right arm straight out to the side parallel to the floor. On an exhalation, turn it inward (or medially), first rotating the thumb down toward the floor, then turning the palm up toward the ceiling with the thumb pointing toward whatever's behind you. Exaggerate the accompanying rounding of the right shoulder, then exhale and swing the forearm behind your torso, parallel to your waist. With your left hand, pull the muscle of the front right armpit (pectoralis major) out of the armpit and lift it up toward the top of the shoulder, then slide your right forearm up your back until it's in the channel of and parallel to the spine.

Next, inhale and reach your left arm straight up toward the ceiling and rotate it outward (laterally), so the palm turns back and the thumb points out to the left. Bend the elbow and reach down for the right hand. Never force yourself to grip the hands. If they don't touch easily, hold a strap between them. Stay in the pose anywhere from 1 to 3 minutes, then release the arms quickly. Return to Fortunate. Repeat for the same length of time with the legs and arms reversed. Finish again in Fortunate.

Traditional Benefit

None listed.

LITTLE LAMP: SANKATA

SANKATA • "brought together," contracted, closed, narrow, strait; crowded together, dense; impervious, impassable; dangerous, critical; difficulty, critical condition, danger to or from

Sankata is a kind of contracted Cow Face legs. This pose is optional.

Practice

From Cow Face, lift your buttocks off the floor and tuck each heel under the opposite buttock.

Traditional Benefit

None listed.

HERO POSE (VIRASANA)

> *VIRA* · a man, especially a brave or eminent man, hero,
> chief (sometimes applied to gods, such as Indra or
> Vishnu); men, people, mankind; heroic, powerful,
> strong, excellent, eminent (compare to the Latin *vir,*
> or "man," from the Proto-Indo-European root *wi-ro,*
> from which come the English "virtue, virile, world,
> virtuoso," and oddly "werewolf")

In its modern incarnation, Hero is similar to Diamond, except that the buttocks are positioned between the feet, either resting on the floor or on a firm support. Gheranda and Svatmarama seem to have different notions about Hero, though it's not clear from any of my sources just what the latter is talking about. I'll offer one interpretation of Svatmarama's Hero as a beginning alternative to Gheranda, then describe Gheranda's Hero for more experienced students.

Gheranda's Hero is the first instance of a Lotus-like position in this sequence, which means you need to be on Lotus Alert for the safety and health of your knees. Have a block handy in case the Lotus knee needs a support. In the modern practice of asana, you might be familiar with

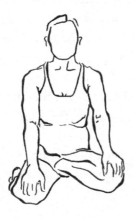

Fig. 12. Hero Pose (*virasana*).

this leg position as the foundation for what's called *bharadvajasana* II (Bharadvaja means "skylark," and is the name of a Vedic sage; see *Light on Yoga* #112).

Practice 1: Svatmarama's Hero

From Fortunate, grab the left ankle and swivel the foot to the outside of the left hip, just as you did for Bull. But don't slide the knee off to the side; keep it aligned with the left hip, perpendicular to the pelvis. Now bring the right leg vertical, stand the foot on the floor, and tuck the heel up by the right buttock. One source shows the left hand resting on the left knee, palm down, and the bent right elbow propped on the right knee, with the chin resting on the right palm. Another source shows the hands resting palms down on their same-side knees.

Stay in this pose for 1 to 3 minutes, then return to Fortunate, taking the left leg out of position as you did for the Frog-like leg in Bull. Repeat with the legs reversed for the same length of time. Return to Fortunate.

Practice 2: Gheranda's Hero

From Fortunate, grab the left ankle and swivel the foot to the outside of the left hip, just as you did for Bull. But don't slide the knee off to the side; keep it aligned with the left hip, perpendicular to the pelvis.

Keeping the knee *completely flexed,* lift the right leg and wedge the outer edge of the foot in the crook of the left elbow. It's common for the foot to be slightly "sickled," that is, turned inward, so press through the inner foot and equalize the lengths of the inner and outer ankles. Rock the leg back and forth, warming up the right hip joint. Now swivel the right leg from the hip and press the outer edge of the foot into the front hip crease of the left leg, keeping the right knee lifted away from the floor. Once the edge of the foot is in place, again swivel from the hip and lower the knee, drawing it as close as you can to the left one.

It's important now *not* to force the right knee to the floor if it doesn't lay there easily at first. If your knee is floating above the floor, support it on a block.

For most of the poses up to now, I've been suggesting your stay be between 1 and 3 minutes. Now that we've inserted a Lotus leg into the equation, the time you stay in this and the other poses in the family will be determined by your experience with Lotus. If you've been working with this pose for a while and it's fairly easy for you, then 1 to 3 minutes is appropriate. But if you're new to Lotus, and especially if you're just learning it from this book without an experienced teacher to supervise your practice, stay no more than 10 seconds at first. This isn't a misprint: swing the Lotus leg into place and then take it pretty much right out again. I'll go into more detail about developing Lotus when I get to the actual pose itself. For now, all you newcomers — 10 seconds and out!

To release the Lotus leg, lift the knee and, still keeping it completely flexed, straighten the leg out to the side. Swing it back in front of your torso from the hip and lay it on the floor. Return to Bull, then repeat Hero with the legs reversed for the same length of time. At the end of Hero, return to Fortunate.

Traditional Benefit
None listed.

Variation
There are a bewildering number of traditional poses named Hero; all are sitting poses except for one standing pose that looks something like Tree. Most of the sitting poses are of the crossed-leg variety, a position pretty well covered by the Perfected Family (see Section 11).

LITTLE LAMP: SANSKRIT ROOTS

A staggering number of English words are related to Sanskrit. We just saw one in the previous pose: our English "cow" can be traced back to the Sanskrit *go* (or *gau*). *Vira* shows up in English in several common words, including "virile," "virtue," and "virtuoso." But it's also hidden in our "world," which, according to the *Dictionary of Word Origins*, originally meant "age of man (*vir*)," or "the course of man's life, of man's experience . . . a chain of senses that culminated in the present sense of the place in which man [and woman] finds himself." Want some more? I could probably fill up the rest of this chapter with examples, so here are just a few common words (and their Sanskrit root): eat (*ad*); eye (*aksha*); divine (*deva*); navy (*nau*, "boat"); night (*nakta*); nose (*nas*); sew (*siv*); video (*vid*); mother (*matri*); and of course, yoga (*yuj*).

Lotus Pose (Padmasana)

PADMA · lotus

Lotus Pose, along with maybe Headstand and Shoulderstand, is one of the most widely recognizable yoga poses. It's impossible to completely understand the liberating effect of this sitting position unless you've experienced the full pose (or at least its halfway modification) for yourself. There's something about the arrangement of the crossed and locked legs that both grounds and lightens the body-mind, spontaneously readying it for conscious breathing or meditation.

But full Lotus, as I've already stated, can be a difficult and potentially injurious pose for the average student. If you're a beginner, I strongly recommend you work first with Half-Lotus Pose (*ardha padmasana*), which is Practice 1 in this section, and only progress to the full pose under the supervision of an experienced teacher. More experienced students with minimal experience with Lotus should begin their stay in the pose with only a few seconds and increase their time very gradually over a few weeks or months, depending on the regularity of their practice.

Svatmarama describes three versions of Lotus, each with a different

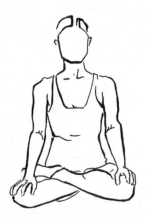

Fig. 13. Lotus Pose (*padmasana*).

placement of the hands and arms. The first is what we call Bound Lotus Pose (*baddha padmasana;* see *Light on Yoga* #55), in which the arms are crossed behind the back torso and the hands catch the same-side feet (which are pressed against the opposite-side groins). This is also Gheranda's version. In the second version, which is also how Anonymous/Shiva describes it, the "upturned hands" (*uttana pani*) rest on the midthighs. In the third version, the hands are cupped (*samputita*) in front of the torso at the level of the navel, one over the other, so the fingers of each hand touch the base of the palm of the other.

LITTLE LAMP: MORE LOTUS NAMES

Lotus has a host of traditional names, including *kamala* ("lotus"); *ambuja* ("produced in water, water born"); *abja* ("born in water"); *amburuha* ("water growing"); *saroruha* ("sitting on a lotus"; a name for Brahma as he sat on a lotus growing from Vishnu's navel).

Practice 1: Half-Lotus

From Staff Pose, cross your shins in front of your torso and sit in an Easy Pose–like position. Bend your right knee and notch the outer edge of the foot in the crook of your left elbow, wrap your right knee in the crook of your right elbow, and hug the foreleg to your chest. Notice if the foot is inverted, meaning the inner ankle is squeezed, while the outer ankle is overstretched. Push through the inner edge of the foot against the upper arm to equalize the lengths of the inner and outer ankles. When you bring the foot across into the left groin, see that you maintain this even stretch of the ankles.

Make sure your right knee is completely flexed, with the back of the thigh and calf in firm contact. Rock the foreleg back and forth a few times. Swiveling *from the hip and not the knee,* snug the outside edge of the foot into the inner left groin. If possible, press the right heel into the left lower belly. Look at the right sole: try to turn the foot so that the plane of the sole is perpendicular (not parallel) to the floor.

This is Half-Lotus. If you're just beginning to practice this pose, stay no more than a few seconds, then release the right leg. Stretch both legs out into Staff, and bounce your knees on the floor a few times. Repeat the pose for the same length of time with the left leg.

Technically, when the right leg is crossed over the left, it's called Right Half-Lotus Pose (*dakshina ardha padmasana*), and when the left is over the right, it's Left Half-Lotus Pose (*vama ardha padmasana*).

Practice 2: Full Lotus

From Half-Lotus, lean back slightly, pick the right leg up off the floor, and lift the left leg in front of the right. To do this, hold the underside of the left shin in your hands. Carefully slide the left leg over the right, snugging the edge of the left foot deep into the right groin. Again, swivel into position from the hip joint, press the left heel against the lower right belly, and arrange the sole perpendicular to the floor. Draw the knees as close together as possible. Use the edges of the feet to press the groins toward the floor, and lift through the top of the sternum. Stay for 1 to 3 minutes, then release the legs into Staff and bounce the knees a few times. Repeat with the legs reversed for the same length of time.

Traditional Benefit

All three sourcebooks claim that Lotus wards off disease. The *Hatha-Yoga-Pradipika* and *Shiva-Samhita* suggest that through working with the breath in Lotus, the practitioner can achieve liberation.

LITTLE LAMP: YOGA

If I read Gheranda correctly, Yoga Pose is a kind of "loose" Lotus. In his directions for the latter, he says to place each foot on top of the opposite thigh (*uru*), while for Yoga, he says to place each foot on the opposite knee (*janu*). This pose is optional.

Practice

Cross each foot over to the opposite thigh, gaze at the tip of the nose, and lay the backs of the hands on the floor outside the hips.

Traditional Benefit

Gheranda makes reference to this pose bringing "success" in yoga.

ROOSTER POSE (KUKKUTASANA)

KUKKUTA · rooster

Full Rooster involves slipping the hands and arms between the Lotus-shaped thighs and calves, pressing the hands to the floor, and lifting the torso and legs off the floor. This is beyond the ability of most students, so here we'll perform a "free-arm" variation of Rooster that today is called Scale Pose (*tolasana*, literally "poising one's self, weighing"; see *Light on Yoga* #48). There are two practices, the first for Half-Lotus and the second for full Lotus. If you have trouble lifting off the floor in either version, press each hand against either the side or the face of a yoga block to create more space between you and the floor.

Practice 1: Scale in Half-Lotus

In Half-Lotus, you may not be able to quite lift the lower leg off the floor. If not, bind the lower leg to the upper one with a strap. Make a loop, pass it under the bottom foot and over the top leg's inner groin, and snug (but don't tighten) it. Press your hands to the floor beside your hips; lean your torso slightly forward; and firming your lower belly, lift your legs off the floor with an exhalation. Hold for 15 to 30 seconds, then lower lightly back down to the floor.

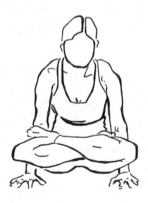

Fig. 14. Rooster Pose (*kukkutasana*).

Practice 2: Scale in Full Lotus

The instructions for Scale in full Lotus are the same as those for Half-Lotus.

Traditional Benefit

None listed.

FISH POSE (MATSYASANA)

MATSYA · fish

Traditionally, Fish Pose might be called Reclining Lotus, because it's performed as a flat-out supine position with the legs in Lotus (see *Light on Yoga* #114). In modern yoga, it's sometimes performed as a backbend with the head and legs on the floor, the arms crossed overhead, and the torso arched off the floor (*Light on Yoga* #113). Here, we'll work with the traditional flat-out version.

If you find it difficult to recline your torso fully on the floor, then you have two choices: you can lie back on some kind of support, such as a bolster or thickly folded blanket, or before you lie back, you can slip your legs out of Half- or full Lotus and simply cross them in Easy Pose (*sukhasana*).

LITTLE LAMP: WHY DOES FISH POSE LOOK LIKE A FISH?

How or why does this pose look like a fish? This question bothered me for a long time, as I assumed that every pose named after a living

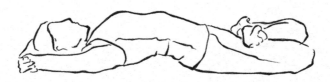

Fig. 15. Fish Pose (*matsyasana*).

creature should look at least vaguely like its namesake. Then I ran across this explanation in *Popular Yoga Asanas* by Swami Kuvalayananda: "The pose is called Matsyasana because in swimming a person can float on water, like the fish, for a considerable time, if he steadily lies there in this posture."[7] It sounds somewhat plausible, though I'm not sure the pose is really needed if all you want to do is float.

This brings up a question: is floating part of traditional Hatha Yoga? It turns out the answer is yes, at least it was 650 years ago in the time of Svatmarama. His instructions are to swallow a large amount of air into your belly and then you can float (*plu*) happily like a lotus leaf, even in deep (*agadha*) water. This is a *pranayama*, believe it or not, called Floating (*plavini*). I suppose this practice might have been akin to our current floating in an isolation tank. By the way, can you swallow air? The answer, again, is yes.

Practice

In Lotus, exhale, lie back, and cross your forearms overhead, holding each elbow with the opposite hand. Stay in position for up to 1 minute. Bring the torso and head up with an inhalation, leading with your chest if possible and letting your head trail.

Traditional Benefit

Fish Pose wards off disease.

LITTLE LAMP: UTTANA KURMASANA

Raised Tortoise Pose is traditionally performed with the arms inserted through the Lotus legs, just like Rooster. But we'll do it with the arms outside the Lotus legs. This pose is optional.

Practice

From Fish, draw the legs in to the torso and wrap the arms around the outer thighs. Stay in this position for one to two minutes.

Traditional Benefit

None listed.

SECTION 5: FORWARD BENDS

There are four poses in this section: one of them an asana-like mudra (*maha mudra*); one a straight-ahead sitting forward bend; one a pose that changed its shape entirely between the time of Svatmarama and that of Gheranda; and the fourth, which isn't a forward bend but the only real twist in *Gheranda-Samhita*.

GREAT SEAL (MAHA MUDRA)

We'll run into Great Seal again as itself in the next chapter. Here we'll use the position as a jumping-off place for a sitting forward bend we call Head-to-Knee Pose (*janu shirshasana*; see *Light on Yoga* #59). I should note that there's been some controversy about this interpretation of the Sanskrit name in certain quarters of the yoga community—not about *janu*, which everyone agrees means "knee" (and cognate with Latin *genu*, from which we get "genuflect"), nor over *shirsha*, which undeniably means "head." The disagreement swirls around the preposition "to," which some believe should be "of," a seemingly slight change with significant implications.

According to the latter camp, the expression "head-*to*-knee" isn't entirely wrong (after all, in the final position of the pose, the practitioner's head is on the straight-leg knee), it just encourages a mistaken idea

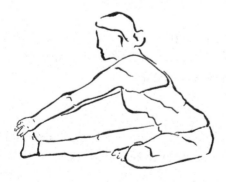

Fig. 16. Great Seal (*maha mudra*).

about the goal of the exercise, especially in beginning students. Hearing "head-to-knee," beginners often take this as a divine command and try, despite their physical limitations such as tight hamstrings, to do just that, resulting in all sorts of strange-looking and potentially injurious forward bends. So the "of" camp maintains that the "head-on-the-top-of-your-shoulders-to-the-straight-knee" is an unstated, distant goal; more to the point, the immediate goal is to press the actual "head of the knee," that is, the kneecap of the *bent knee* away from the pelvis to trigger the forward bend. This is a well-known movement in Bound Angle Pose, which we performed earlier in the sequence as Fortunate Pose, except that it involves both knees simultaneously pressing *away* from the pelvis (but not *down* toward the floor). It's supposed to center the heads of the thigh-bones and so help release the torso into a forward bend. This same logic is now being applied to Head-to-Knee Pose, its bent knee being the equivalent of one *baddha konasana* knee.

Which of the two interpretations is correct? Let's just say that both make sense. The more common "to-the-knee" interpretation does suggest at least an ultimate though not ultimately important goal. What's more important for everyone, beginner and more experienced student, in the forward bend is to keep the front torso as long as possible and not to bend forward from the belly. The "of-the-knee" interpretation will indeed assist the more inflexible beginners and ensure that they don't get the wrong idea about the performance of Head-to-Knee Pose.

Have a strap handy for this practice, and if you're more flexible, a block as well.

Practice

Sit on your support in Staff Pose. Bend your left knee and bring the heel to your perineum, then lay the leg on the floor. If it doesn't rest there easily, support it on a block or folded blanket, but don't let the knee float unsupported. If you're less flexible, arrange the left shin perpendicular to the right leg; if you're more flexible, draw the bent leg into a somewhat-greater-than-90-degree angle. Turn your torso to the right. Wrap the strap around your right sole, hold it in your left hand, and press your right hand to the floor outside your right hip. Keeping your torso vertical, walk your left hand along the strap until your arm is perfectly straight.

Take a few breaths, pulling on the strap with your left hand and pressing against the floor with your right, and intensify your torso's right twist. Exhale and swing your right hand to the outside half of the strap (that is, the part of the strap to the outside of the right leg), and hold the inside half in your left hand. Grip the strap firmly, lift your torso, and *push the head of your left knee away from the hip,* using that movement to anchor your pelvis. Ideally, this movement will initiate a forward release of the torso; when it does, slacken your grip on the strap and, exhaling, *lightly* walk your hands forward along the strap for a few inches, then stop. Inhale, pull on the strap, and lift the front torso (or spine if you prefer to think of it that way); on another exhalation, walk your hands lightly along the strap a few more inches. Remember not to pull yourself forcefully into a forward bend, and keep your elbows straight as you walk your hands along the strap. Continue in this fashion until you feel a comfortable stretch in the backs of your legs or until you begin to round forward from your belly. Then stop and hold the strap. Try to create some space in the groins to allow the forward bend to deepen.

Stay in the pose for 1 to 3 minutes. If you can comfortably hold the sides of your right foot, put one face of the block against your sole and reach out farther for the block's back side to keep your arms as long as possible. Remember: never force your head down on the straight-leg knee. Come up with an inhalation, return to neutral Staff, and repeat the pose with the opposite leg for the same length of time. Finish by returning to Staff one more time.

Traditional Benefit

The traditional benefit is listed under the Great Seal (*maha mudra*) in chapter 6.

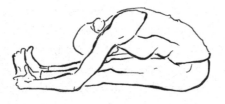

Fig. 17. Intense-Stretch-of-the-West Pose (*pashchima uttanasana*).

INTENSE-STRETCH-OF-THE-WEST POSE (PASHCHIMA UTTANASANA)

PASHCHIMA · last, final; West

UT · intense

TAN · extend, stretch

Intense-Stretch-of-the-West Pose (*pashchima uttanasana;* hereafter referred to as West) is the familiar sitting forward bend. Nothing much has changed about it for more than five hundred years. In his asana chapter, Gheranda describes this pose in four easy steps: sit on the floor, stretch your legs out like sticks (*dandas*), hold your feet with your hands, and put your forehead on your shins. We'll practice with a little more attention to detail.

Practice

There's no secret to the performance of West. Sit on the floor or a support of an appropriate height, and stretch your legs out through your heels. Press your hands against the floor beside your hips and lift your chest in Staff Pose. I'll describe two ways of moving into West: the first is for stiffer, beginning students, who will need to use a yoga strap, and the second is for more experienced, flexible students, for whom the strap is optional.

Whether you're using the strap or holding your feet, it's important to come down into the forward bend from your groins, not your belly. Remember first of all that if you're using the strap, your feet aren't the goal in this pose.

Never force yourself into a forward bend, especially when sitting on the floor. Coming forward, as soon as you feel the length between your pubis and navel shortening, stop, lift up slightly, and lengthen the space again. Often, because of tightness in the backs of the legs, a beginner's forward bend doesn't go very far forward and might look more like a "sitting-up-straight" pose.

Practice 1: For Beginners

Sit on a support of an appropriate height in Staff and wrap a strap around your soles. Hold the strap firmly in both hands, with your arms long and your torso upright (perpendicular to the floor). When you're ready to bring the torso forward, slacken your grip on the strap and, with an exhalation, walk your hands lightly along the strap for a few inches. Stop, grip the strap again, inhale, and lift your chest. Now exhale, slacken your grip again, and walk your hands lightly along the strap for a few more inches. Continue in this fashion until you either (1) start to bend forward from your belly — at which point stop, back off the strap a few inches, and lift your chest to lengthen your front torso — or (2) are comfortably able to hold the sides of your feet.

Practice 2: For Intermediates

If you're more flexible and can lean forward from the groins with a long front spine, then you can hold the sides of your feet. If you're less flexible though, please use a strap to wrap around your soles, and start with your torso upright and arms straight and proceed according to the instructions for Practice 1.

Traditional Benefit

Oddly, Gheranda has nothing to say about the benefits of West, but Svatmarama waxes eloquent. He calls West the "foremost" or "best" (*agrya*) among the asanas. He says it causes the "purifier" breath (*pavana*) to flow through the "back" or "west" (*pashchima*), by which I assume he means the *sushumna nadi*. It stokes the "fire in the belly" (*jathara anala*), tones the belly (*udara*), and brings good health (*maroga*, literally "not disease").

Cautions

I want to emphasize the need to sit high enough in this deep forward bend. The pelvis has to tip forward to protect the back. If you're sitting too low, that won't happen, and as a result, the lower back will be overstretched, possibly leading to strain.

Variation

You can perform West lying on your back. This is not, remember, like the modern Plow Pose (*halasana*), in which the torso is braced on the tops of the shoulders and the torso is perpendicular to the floor. In this variation, traditionally and aptly called Sleeping Intense-Stretch-of-the-West Pose (*shayita pashchima uttanasana*), as much of the back torso as possible is on the floor. Nowadays this pose is called Face-Upward Intense-Stretch-of-the-West Pose (*urdhva mukha pashchima uttanasana*; see *Light on Yoga* #70).

LITTLE LAMP: EAST IS EAST AND WEST IS WEST — DIRECTIONS IN PRACTICE

> Space, the substratum of the cosmos, is the abode, the source, of all forms. Hence the directions, the determinants of space, have a special significance. Particular powers or deities are symbolically connected with the directions of space, the nature of which they reveal and express.
>
> —Alain Danielou, *The Gods of India,* 129

What direction do you face when you practice yoga? You probably don't think about this much, but for the ancient Hindus, the cardinal and intermediate points of the compass had, as Alain Danielou writes, a "special significance." Each of the eight points was watched over by an armed god, or "world protector" (*loka pala*), who stood for a particular beneficent quality. For example, the east was guarded by the thunderbolt-wielding Indra, considered the lord of all the protectors and the prototype of courage and power.

The symbolism of these directions played an important role in many aspects of Indian life. In the *Chandogya-Upanishad,* there's an account of the traditional newborn-naming rite. The father holds the child and turns to each cardinal point, pausing to petition the reigning deity for the child's protection, concluding with the fervent hope, "May I never make mourning for a son!" (3.15.2; translation by Valerie Roebuck). On the other end of life's journey, the ritual honoring deceased ancestors was always performed facing south, the region of Yama, the god of the dead. (In the Occident, the land of departed spirits is situated to the west. Remember how Frodo and Gandalf sailed into the setting sun at the end of the *Lord of the Rings* trilogy?)

Yogis were enjoined to face in one of two symbolic directions. "Let him go to a pure place," writes the sage Shankara in his commentary to the *Yoga-Sutra,* and "take his seat (*asana*), facing east or north" (translation by Trevor Leggett). East is the quarter of the rising sun, a worldwide symbol of the source of all earthly life and the "dawn" of spiritual insight. North is the quarter of the polestar, the fixed hub around which the starry universe rotates, and a symbol of our own center, the Self.

LITTLE LAMP: *PASHCHIMA*

It seems surprising that Svatmarama praises West as the "foremost" (*agrya*) among the asanas. Why the ringing endorsement for what seems to us a simple hamstring stretch? Apparently, according to Svatmarama, West is much more than that. It stokes the "fire in the belly" or digestive juices (*jathara anala*), firms the belly, and gives us good health— believable enough and certainly worthy of recognition. We need to go back to the first chapter of the *Gheranda-Samhita* to find out how to do this stoking, where Gheranda tells us to move the "lower belly" (*vasti*) gently (*shana*) while contracting the anus (*payu*).

We still have to wonder, though, if improved digestion and a trim waistline qualify this pose as the best. It turns out that what's really important is the effect the fire in the belly has on our dormant vital energy, here called *pavana.* Svatmarama claims West encourages the *pavana* to flow in the West (*pashchima*). In the yoga lexicon, "west" usually refers to the entire back of the body—just as the "east" (*purva*) is the front— so the name of the pose (West) tells us which side of us is exposed and where to expect the stretch (*tan*) in the forward bend. But West has a double meaning here. It refers not only to the back of the physical body but also to the *sushumna nadi,* the subtle central conduit located in the back body and following the course of the physical spine from the tailbone to the atlas and then on to the crown. This pose then, according to Svatmarama, plays a significant role in directing the body's vital energy into *sushumna,* one of the final goals of Hatha Yoga. I'll go into this in more detail in chapter 8.

BOW POSE (DHANURASANA) 1
SVATMARAMA'S VERSION

DHANU · bow (from *dhanv,* "to go" or "to kill")

In 1350, Svatmarama's Bow Pose (*dhanurasana*) is a sitting pose, what today we call Toward-the-Ear Bow Pose (*akarna dhanurasana,* see *Light on Yoga* #173). This position approximates an archer, presumably a warrior, wielding a bow, the arm and hand holding the straight-leg big toe (figuratively holding the bow's grip) and the other hand pulling the other foot's big toe near the ear, representing the drawn arrow. Three hundred years later, Gheranda applied the same name to the eponymous backbend with which most of us are familiar—the torso and legs representing the upper and lower limbs of the bow and the arms its string. Here we have an example of the same name being applied to different poses, and a change in images from someone *using* a bow to someone *being* the bow itself.

Have a strap handy for this exercise.

Practice

Start from West. If you're in a full forward bend, grip the big toes with the same-side index and middle fingers, secured with the thumbs; on an inhalation, straighten your arms and lift your torso as much as possible. Now bend your left knee, swivel your torso open slightly to the left, and with another inhalation, draw the left foot to (or toward) your left ear.

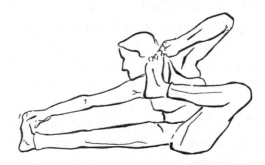

Fig. 18. Bow Pose (*dhanurasana*) 1—Svatmarama's version.

If you're using a strap in West, take it in your right hand. Bend your left knee, put the foot on the floor, and then grip the big toe with your left index and middle fingers, secured with the thumb. Swivel your torso open slightly to the left and, with an inhalation, lift your left foot toward your left ear. If you need to use a strap to hold the straight-leg foot, you may also need the support of a chair or block for the raised foot. Position the block or chair to the outside of the left hip, then rest the left heel on the top end of the block or the chair seat.

This version of Bow is one of the few instances of a true sidebend in modern asana, which means the side torso on the straight-leg side will shorten or compress as much as possible, and the raised-leg side will lengthen or round as much as possible. Look out over the straight leg as if you were Arjuna, the great warrior in the *Bhagavad-Gita,* gazing at a bull's-eye. Hold this position anywhere from 30 seconds to a minute, then straighten the bent leg and return to West. Repeat to the opposite side for the same length of time. Finish back in Staff Pose.

Traditional Benefit
None listed.

Variation
Gheranda's version of Bow is found in Section 6.

LITTLE LAMP: *DHANU*

The bow is a well-known symbol in the yoga tradition. Along with the arrow and armor, it's typically associated with the warrior, who in turn stands for the yogi battling against the forces of self-ignorance (*avidya*). In the *Mundaka-Upanishad* (Shaved Head Upanishad; 2.2.3–4), the bow, arrow, and target are three elements in a kind of spiritual target practice. The bow stands for both the collective wisdom of the Upanishads and that wisdom's concentrated "seed" (*bija*), the mantra OM. The arrow, which is propelled by the bow-mantra, is the embodied self (*atman*), "sharpened by meditation," and the arrow's target or bull's-eye is the great self (*parama atman*).

The bow and arrow images are used differently in the *Maitri-Upanishad* (Benevolent Upanishad; 6.28). Despite its reputation as a force for non-violence, there are nevertheless many images in yoga of killing off what are considered the undesirable parts of our psyche. Here the bow (or its string) is the yogi; the arrow is "freedom from self-conceit," which is used to "slay" unwanted attributes, such as greed, envy, sloth, and impurity, that block our way to self-realization.

Lord of Fish Pose (Matsyendrasana)

MATSYA · fish

INDRA · lord (in Sanskrit, when the initial *i* of one word follows the concluding *a* of another, the two letters blend into an *e*; hence, *matysa + indra = matsyendra*)

Lord of Fish Pose is the lone twist in both the *Hatha-Yoga-Pradipika* and *Gheranda-Samhita*. In the modern school of Iyengar Yoga, there are four variations of this pose: the first three are designated as "half" (*ardha*) and followed by a Roman numeral (I, II, or III); the fourth is called "full" (*paripurna*) and unnumbered, this most likely being Iyengar's interpretation of Svatmarama's instruction. I'm not a Sanskritist, so I can't comment directly on the clarity of Gheranda's instruction for this pose, but the translations in my several sourcebooks are all rather confusing. If I

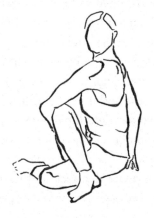

Fig. 19. Lord of Fish Pose (*matsyendrasana*).

didn't already know what Lord of Fish looked like, I'd have a hard time figuring out what to do from the available English renditions.

It seems fairly clear that in *Hatha-Yoga-Pradipika* and *Gheranda-Samhita,* the foot of the leg we twist away from (that is, the leg that rests on the floor) is in Half-Lotus. This is what Iyengar does for half variations II and III and the full pose. We'll work instead with a leg position similar to Iyengar's first half variation (*ardha matsyendrasana* I, #116), in which the foot is brought to the outside of the opposite hip (actually, Iyengar *sits* on that foot).

Practice

From Staff, bend your knees and rest your feet on the floor, heels about a foot from your buttocks. Slide the left foot under the right knee to the outside of the right hip and lay the bent left leg on the floor. See that your left knee is on an imaginary line drawn out from your navel, perpendicular to your torso. Now step your right foot to the floor outside your left thigh, and draw your right heel as close to your left hip as possible. Just to be clear, the right leg is now vertical, with the knee pointing toward the ceiling.

Exhale and rotate your torso to the right. Gheranda instructs us to press the left elbow against the right knee, cup the chin in the right palm, and gaze between the eyebrows. It might be more useful, however, to wrap your left arm around your right leg, and press your right hand on the floor behind your pelvis. It's possible you've seen this pose performed with the arm pressed against the *outside* of the knee, but most of us have to hunch over to get into that position, which interferes with the twist. I strongly recommend that you wrap the leg with the arm.

Now lean your torso back slightly and draw your belly up and in (just as Gheranda says to do), then hug your inner thigh to your belly. Press the inner right foot (the mound of the big toe and inner heel) firmly to the floor, and at the same time, release the outer right hip downward. As you press the inner foot, soften the inner right groin, and from the depth of the groin, lift your navel up along the inner thigh.

The natural tendency in this pose is to rotate the neck and head in the same direction as the torso, but I like to rotate them in the opposite direction; if you'd like to try this, rotate your head to the left and look over your left shoulder. Stay in this pose for a minute, release back to the beginning bent-knee position, reverse the legs, and repeat to the left for the same length of time. Now get ready for backbends.

Traditional Benefit

Gheranda is silent on the benefits of Lord of Fish, but Svatmarama gushes. Like all twists, Lord of Fish stokes the "fire in the belly" (*jathara pradipta*) and so helps destroy disease and contributes to the awakening of the *kundalini*.

Caution

If you have any problems with or injuries to your neck, don't turn your head in either direction—keep it in a neutral position.

LITTLE LAMP: HOW A FISH BECAME A LORD

Once upon a time, there was a fisherman who lived in Kamarupa on the shore of the Ita sea. One day while he was fishing, a huge fish snagged his line, and though he tugged with all his might on the fishing pole, he was dragged into the water and swallowed by the fish. Luckily, his good karma saved him from being digested.

Right about the same time, the goddess Uma ("helper, friend, companion") was asking Mahadeva ("great god"; that is, Shiva) for instruction in yoga. Shiva said, "This information has to be kept secret, so to be on the safe side, let's build a house under the ocean and do the teaching there." So they built their submarine abode, and Shiva began his talk. But even though she had asked for the teaching, it wasn't long before Uma dozed off; Shiva, unaware of this, continued on with his exposition. He would have been talking to himself, but it seems that the fish with our fisherman in its belly was floating nearby, and the fisherman heard every word. So when Shiva asked Uma if she understood, not realizing yet she was fast asleep, the now-enlightened fisherman unthinkingly replied, "Yes, I understand." Of course, Shiva thought it was his wife who had answered.

Just as Shiva finished speaking, Uma awoke. Realizing she'd fallen asleep during the teaching, she asked Shiva to start again from about the middle. Shiva was confused. "I thought you said you understood," he said to Uma, who smiled.

"No, dear," she explained, "that rough night I had last night caught up with me, and I feel asleep about thirty minutes ago."

Shiva was now really confused. "Well," he said, "then who said, 'I understand'?"

Uma shrugged. "Wasn't me."

Shiva looked around, but in a house under the sea, there aren't many intruders. Then he switched on his "third eye," equivalent to Superman's X-ray vision, and lo and behold, he spied our fisherman in the fish's belly. There was nothing for Shiva to do now but initiate our fisherman, who then spent the next twelve years meditating in the fish's belly. Then one day, another fisherman caught our fisherman's fish, and bringing it to his boat thought, "This fish is so heavy, maybe there's a treasure in its belly." So he eagerly cut the belly open, expecting gold and silver, but instead found our enlightened fisherman.

Assuming the name Minapa ("fish"), or in some versions, Matsyendra ("lord of fish"), he's remembered today as the human progenitor of Hatha Yoga.

SECTION 6: BACKBENDS

There are either four or five backbends in the Original sequence, depending on how you decide to treat Sea Monster Pose (*makarasana*). Compared to many modern backbends, these are all fairly easy exercises. They are found exclusively in the *Gheranda-Samhita*.

General Caution

If you're dealing with a back or neck injury, you should consult with an experienced teacher before tackling any backbend. If your neck is sore for whatever reason, then don't extend it (that is, take your head back toward your back torso) or look up when you lift your upper torso and head off the floor; instead, keep your head in a relatively neutral position relative to your shoulders and look down at the floor. You might even support your forehead on a rolled-up blanket or foam block to avoid any strain to your neck.

Sea Monster Pose (Makarasana)

MAKARA · a kind of sea monster (sometimes confused with crocodile, shark, or dolphin)

This pose is often called the Dolphin or Crocodile Pose, but actually a *makara* is one of those wonderfully imaginative hybrid Indian creatures with (according to unsubstantiated reports of sightings) four lion- or dog-like legs, a crocodile or fish tail and scaly body, and an elephant's trunk. We'll use Sea Monster primarily as a resting pose between backbends, though I'll describe a backbend variation you may perform if desired.

Little Lamp: Will the Real Makara Please Stand Up?

There seems to be a small but nevertheless significant difference of opinion about the performance of this exercise between my traditional sources and Iyengar's version. The former picture Sea Monster as described in the following practice. But Iyengar takes Gheranda's instruction to "hold the head in the arms" differently (see *Light on Yoga* #26). He cups the hands on the back of the head, raises the head off the floor, and "holds"or lightly presses the forearms against the sides of the head. He also raises the legs off the floor as in Locust. So what is traditionally more or less a resting pose becomes a "baby backbend" in Iyengar's

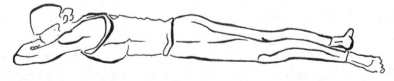

Fig. 20. Sea Monster Pose (*makarasana*).

book. Gheranda says nothing about lifting the upper torso, head, or legs, so it seems likely that Iyengar's Sea Monster is a modern variant of the traditional model. Incidentally, Gheranda has a marvelous word for "arms"—*karadanda*, literally the "hand sticks."

Practice

Lie prone (facedown) on the floor. Separate your legs to about the width of your sticky mat (or even a bit wider), and lay your inner feet on the floor so the toes point out to the sides. Cross your forearms and hold the opposite elbow with each hand. Rest your forehead on your crossed arms, or nestle your head down into the space between your shoulders and your forearms. Stay anywhere from 1 to 3 minutes.

Traditional Benefit

Sea Monster stokes the body's digestive fire (*deha agni*).

Variation

Here's a variation that's somewhere between the traditional pose and Iyengar's version. Instead of resting your head on your crossed forearms, lift your head off the floor, join the bases of your palms with the elbows on the floor shoulder-width apart, and cradle your chin on your open palms.

SERPENT POSE (BHUJANGASANA)

> **BHUJANGA** · serpent, snake (from *bhuj*, "to curve, make crooked")

Often called Cobra Pose, *bhujanga* more properly means "serpent" or "snake." The pose is similar to what we call Upward-Facing Dog Pose (*urdhva mukha shvanasana*), except in Serpent, the fronts of the legs and top feet are pressed to the floor, while in Upward Dog, the legs are off the floor. Serpent can be something of a problematic pose, because in using the hands and arms to lift the torso and head off the floor with the legs pressed against the floor, we tend to push back into and compress the lower spine. Obviously this is something to avoid as much as possible. Please read the following instructions carefully before attempting the full pose. I've divided the practice into three steps; don't move to step 2 until you're comfortable in step 1, and likewise, don't go to step 3 until you understand step 2.

Practice 1: Beginning

Lie in Sea Monster. Slide your legs together, and lift your head and upper torso off the floor, supporting yourself with your forearms on the floor. Set your elbows directly below your shoulders so your upper arms are perpendicular to the floor, and your forearms parallel to each other. Spread your palms, and press the bases of your index fingers into the floor. Press the tops of your feet into the floor as well, making sure your little toes are in contact with the floor. The latter movement, created by turning the thighs slightly inward (medially), tends to push the tailbone toward the ceiling. Counter this by firming the tail against the back pelvis.

This is what we'll call step 1 of the pose, and you may feel most comfortable staying in this position. Hold for 30 seconds to 1 minute, then release with an exhalation back to Sea Monster. You might want to repeat the pose once or twice more.

Practice 2: Intermediate

If you're comfortable in step 1, then move on to step 2. Now you can lift your elbows a few inches off the floor, but don't straighten them completely yet. This seems simple enough, but there's a trick involved. As I mentioned earlier, our tendency here is to lift the head and torso higher

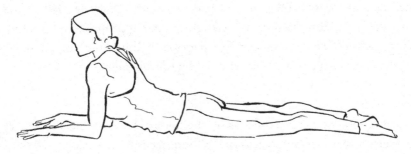

Fig. 21. Serpent Posture (*bhujangasana*), step 2.

by pushing into and compressing the lower back. So as you lift your elbows, be sure to move your sternum and tailbone in *opposite* directions: the former should ideally move *forward* toward the front edge of your sticky mat; the latter should lengthen *backward* toward your heels. This helps keep the lower spine long even though it's moving toward a deep extension.

Again, decide what's best for you: do you stay here or move on? If you're staying, hold for 30 seconds to 1 minute, then release with an exhalation back to Sea Monster. You might want to repeat the pose once or twice more.

Practice 3: Full Pose

If you can keep the lower back relatively long and all feels well, then you can move on to step 3. With an inhalation, slowly straighten your elbows, still moving the sternum and tailbone in opposite directions. Support the lift of the sternum by firming the shoulder blades against the back torso, but avoid pushing the front ribs forward. Take your head back a bit, but keep your shoulders down away from your ears. When the belly is pressed against the floor as it is in this pose, its movement is restricted, which can make breathing difficult. Be sure to direct your breath into your back torso.

Hold the pose anywhere from 30 seconds to a minute, breathing easily. Release back to Sea Monster with an exhalation. If you like, you can repeat the pose once or twice more for equal or shorter lengths of time.

Traditional Benefit

Gheranda is extremely enthusiastic about Serpent. He says it increases or augments (*vardha*) the "body's [digestive] fire" (*deha agni*), destroys disease (*roga*, "breaking up of strength"), and appropriately wakes up (*jagarti*) the "serpent goddess" (*bhujagi devi*). This is the only mention in the asana chapter of a pose stimulating the *kundalini*.

Variation

It's also possible to raise the legs off the floor in Serpent, but this makes it even more important to firm the tailbone against the back pelvis, since the raised legs will tend to compress the lower back.

146

For another variation, lie in Sea Monster and clasp your hands behind your back, your thumbs resting on your sacrum. With an inhalation, slide your thumbs along the back of your pelvis toward your feet, and lift your upper torso and head as you would for Serpent. Now lift your arms away from the back of your torso until they're parallel to the floor. Hold the position for 30 seconds to a minute, then release your torso and head back to the floor with an exhalation. Unclasp your hands, and lay your arms on the floor alongside your torso.

LITTLE LAMP: *KUNDALINI*

KUNDALA · ring, bracelet, fetter

What is *kundalini*? That's a good question, the full answer to which is the subject of its own book. To me, *kundalini* is the heroine of a fairy tale the yogis tell to explain something inexplicable, full of dragons and wizards and magic and a holy quest up the side of a mountain. It's like the story of the two Hobbits, Frodo and Sam, except in reverse: they climbed Mount Doom to destroy a ring; we climb Mount Meru to complete one. In this tale, we play two roles, that of the quester, *kundalini,* and the object of her quest—we're the goal of our own search. But before we can begin our ascent, we have to wake the "sleeping princess," coiled round herself at the foot of Meru. In this condition, she represents the slumber of our own self-ignorance. Paradoxically—and ironically—she's both the fetter that binds us to suffering and death and the means of our release from that suffering and attainment of eternal life. What does it take to do this? The application of concentrated and intensified life energy, usually dissipated in amusing or distracting but otherwise unliberating pursuits. Energy so prepared serves as a wake-up call and provides the sustenance for the princess's arduous climb ahead. As she scales Meru, she passes through a half-dozen "stations," each one supplying her with new insights and ammunition for the remaining heights. When she (we) reaches the summit, she meets her other half—us again—from whom her separation, the cause of so much unhappiness, is seen to have been an illusion; she—we—was never really split off from the other.

Innate within us then we each carry the promise of our own fulfill-ment. We must awaken it first, which admittedly takes some effort and commitment and, most of all, courage. We all need a bit of courage to make needed changes in our behavior or personality, but to transform ourselves takes enormous courage and what the yogis call *mumukshu* ("eager to be free, striving after emancipation"). Why hasn't this hap-pened for you yet? That's a question you'll have to ask yourself.

LOCUST POSE (SHALABHASANA)

SHALABHA • grasshopper, locust

Most students are probably familiar with the modern version of Locust, in which the head and upper torso, arms, and feet and legs are raised, leaving only the lower belly touching the floor, so the body assumes the shape of a shallow bowl. This isn't, however, how Gheranda describes the pose. In his traditional version, the palms are pressed to the floor beside the chest, and depending on how you read the brief instruction, there are two possible ways of performing this exercise.

You can raise the upper torso, head, and legs off the floor so that, as with the modern version, the body looks like a shallow bowl. The essen-tial difference between this pose and its modern counterpart is that the hands are pressing the floor, the bent elbows alongside the torso. We'll call this Locust 1.

Alternatively, you can keep the upper chest and chin on the floor and raise the lower body from the navel down off the floor. This version, which we'll call Locust 2, is obviously a bit more challenging.

Practice: Locust 1

Lie in Sea Monster. Slide your legs nearly together, and press your palms, elbows bent, to the floor on either side of your chest, fingers pointing forward. Remember to turn your little toes down to the floor to rotate your thighs inward, and firm your buttocks so your coccyx presses to-ward your pubis. On an inhalation, lift your head, upper torso, and legs off the floor. Try to rely more on the back muscles to lift the torso than the push of the hands on the floor; in fact, don't push the hands against the floor at all to assist the lift. If you have difficulty holding your head and upper torso off the floor in this pose, support your sternum on a rolled-up blanket.

Hold for 30 seconds to 1 minute, then release with an exhalation. If you like, you can repeat once or twice more for equal or shorter lengths of time.

LITTLE LAMP: HOW HIGH?

An interesting question arises here: how high off the floor do we lift the legs? It only comes up because, for all the vagueness of Gheranda's truncated instructions, he's very specific here. But my sources, as often happens, have different ideas about what Gheranda is telling us to do. Two say 9 inches; another says 10 (both unlikely at face value, since there were no "inches" in India in 1650); and the remaining two say 1 cubit, which is, as best as I can discover, an ancient measure somewhere between 17 and 22 inches. Of course, this is a Western cubit, which was the distance between the elbow and the stretched-out middle finger (*cubitum* means "elbow" in Latin). An estimate I found online puts the Indian cubit at around 18 inches.

So digging into the verse itself, it turns out that Gheranda is actually saying to lift the legs a *vitasti,* which equals 12 *angulas,* which is in turn the distance from the tip of the stretched-out thumb to the tip of the little finger. This explains the two measurements given in inches: the distance between these two fingertips on my hand is exactly 9 inches; the 10-inch estimate must have been made by a writer with big hands.

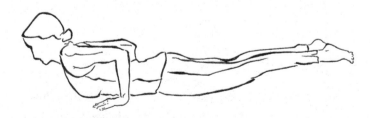

Fig. 22. Locust Pose (*shalabhasana*).

Practice: Locust 2

We'll break this pose into two stages—A and B. For both stages, set yourself up as you did in Locust 1. Here, though, keep the chin and chest on the floor. With an inhalation, press your hands firmly to the floor and lift your right leg as high as you can. Hold for 30 seconds, then release with an exhalation. Repeat with your left leg for the same length of time. This is Locust 2A.

Locust 2B is, obviously, the same as 2A except that both legs are raised at the same time. Again, perform this movement with an inhalation, hold for 20 to 30 seconds, then release with an exhalation back to Sea Monster.

Traditional Benefit

None listed.

Variation

The *Yoga-Rahasya,* attributed to Nathamuni, shows Locust with the head, upper torso, legs, and arms raised, the latter stretched out in front of the torso parallel to the floor.

Bow Pose (Dhanurasana) 2
Gheranda's version

DHANU · bow

As I mentioned in Section 5 regarding to Svatmarama's Bow Pose, by Gheranda's time, the same name was applied to the backbend we're all familiar with today.

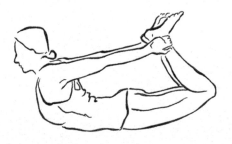

Fig. 23. Bow Pose (*dhanurasana*) 2— Gheranda's version.

Practice

Lie in Sea Monster. Bend your knees, grip your ankles with your hands, and draw your heels toward your buttocks. If you find it difficult to grip your ankles directly, then hold a strap looped around them. To begin, inhale, pull your heels away from your buttocks — keeping your thighs on the floor — and lift your upper torso and head. Hold for 30 seconds to a minute, then release with an exhalation. You can either continue to hold your ankles or return to Sea Monster. Try to pause no longer than about 15 seconds, then inhale and again lift your upper torso and head as you pull your heels off your buttocks. This time, raise your thighs a few inches off the floor. Hold again for 30 seconds to a minute, and this time (if you didn't do so before) release back to Sea Monster. Over the years, I've been taught two balance points for the full pose: either the pubic bone or the navel. Over time, as you practice Gheranda's Bow, work with both points and see which suits you best.

Traditional Benefit

None listed.

CAMEL POSE (USHTRASANA)

USHTRA · camel

Just as traditional Locust is different from its modern incarnation, modern Camel doesn't look much like its predecessor. In fact, traditional Camel looks more like Gheranda's Bow Pose than a camel.

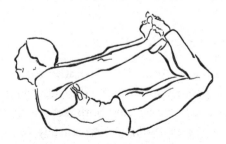

Fig. 24. Camel Pose (*ushtrasana*).

Practice

Camel is very similar to Gheranda's Bow. With the knees bent, simply cross the ankles and hold the opposite-side foot in each hand. Perform the pose as you did Bow, in two stages. Once again, if you find it difficult to grip your ankles directly, then hold a strap looped around them.

Traditional Benefit

None listed.

LITTLE LAMP: SAME NAME, DIFFERENT POSE

We've now run across several examples of traditional and modern poses that have the same name but are performed moderately or wildly differently: in the former category are Lion, Cow Face, Hero, and Locust; in the latter are Tortoise, Garuda, and Camel. Modern yoga has either added some additional element to the traditional shape or invented a new shape entirely.

What about tradition itself? Did something like this happen way back when? Certainly we have the example of the two Bow Poses: Svatmarama's forward-bending version, which looks like an archer drawing a bow, and Gheranda's backbending version, which looks like the bow itself. In Tortoise too, Svatmarama seems to be instructing us to sit on crossed ankles, while Anonymous/Gheranda wants us to evert our feet and sit on the outer heels.

Apparently this "same name, different pose" trend (as well as its opposite, "different pose, same name") isn't at all uncommon in the annals of asana. I found many, many examples in *The Encyclopedia of Traditional Asana.*

SECTION 7: STANDING POSES

Standing poses are few and far between in traditional Hatha Yoga (see the Little Lamp in the Tree Pose practice for more on this subject). I'm including Superior Pose (*utkatasana*) here because both feet are on the floor, so it's similar to standing pose even though it's technically a squat.

It's possible, though, that Superior could be integrated into the sequence in Section 2, following Diamond and just before Lion. I'll go into this more in Appendix 1.

SUPERIOR POSE (UTKATASANA)

> *UTKATA* • exceeding the usual measure, immense, gigantic; richly endowed with, abounding in; drunk, mad, furious; excessive, much; superior, high, proud, haughty; uneven; difficult

You may remember from chapter 3 that the first limb of Gheranda's yoga consists of the six purifying acts (*shat karma shodhana*), which are actually a collection of about twenty different practices that house-clean every nook and cranny of the physical body. One of these twenty is called Wet Bladder (*jala basti* or *vasti*, "lower belly"), in which the practitioner cleans out the anus (*payu*) while squatting in water up to the navel. What's this got to do with Superior? The traditional pose is the preferred position for *jala basti*. It's performed as a full squat with the weight on the balls of the feet and the buttocks resting on the raised heels (see *Gheranda-Samhita* 1.45), presumably in a quick-flowing river. I'm sure you'll be relieved to know that our interest in this pose is purely as an asana, and we won't be practicing it in a river with the help of a thin pipe.

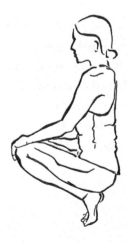

Fig. 25. Superior Pose (*utkatasana*).

LITTLE LAMP: MODERN SUPERIOR

You might be familiar with the modern version of Superior, which is a kind of half-squat with the heels pressed firmly to the floor, the torso leaned slightly forward over the thighs, and the arms stretched overhead (see *Light on Yoga* #17). It's often called Chair Pose, because it looks like the yogi's about to sit down on (or is just getting up from) a chair, but as you can see from the preceding translation, *utkata* doesn't literally mean "chair." The traditional version is slightly different than its modern incarnation.

As you'll soon discover, the balance in this position can indeed be uneven or difficult. There's a short-term solution to any difficulty you might experience. Have a yoga block or two handy, which can be used to brace the knees if needed.

Practice

Stand with your feet hip-width apart, inner feet parallel. With an exhalation, simultaneously bend your knees and raise your heels off the floor, taking your weight on the balls of your feet. Slowly descend into a squat, finally resting your buttocks on your raised heels, with your torso upright. If you have your balance, you won't need a block. But if you find yourself teetering, then put your block (turned on its side) below your knees and use it to brace them.

You can rest your hands on your thighs; press your palms together in *anjali mudra;* or bend your elbows, hold your upper arms beside your torso, reach your forearms forward and parallel to the floor, and make your hands into fists. This last pose, according to one source,[8] is used for milking cows and so is called Milking Cows Pose (*godohikasana*). Stay in the squat for 1 to 2 minutes (with or without a cow), then inhale and straighten your knees, press your heels to the floor, and stand up straight.

Traditional Benefit

None listed.

Caution

As with all flexed-knee poses, be especially careful with your inner knees. If you feel any pain in your knee(s), squat with a thinly rolled blanket between your thighs and calves, or avoid the traditional version of Superior Pose altogether and work with the modern version instead.

Variation

There are many variations of Superior Pose; here are just a few. From Superior, lower your knees to the floor, then spread them wide as in Frog. From Frog, shift your weight onto your left heel, then extend your right leg forward, pressing your heel to the floor. Bring the right foot back and repeat with the left.

TREE POSE (VRIKSHASANA)

> VRIKSHA · any tree and other plants (properly any tree
> bearing flowers and fruit, but can be loosely applied to any
> tree, as well as other plants; possibly connected with *brh*,
> "to grow" or "to root up")

Tree Pose is one of the most familiar standing poses, standard fare in just about every asana class. Here we have another flip-a-coin instruction from Gheranda. He tells us to place the raised foot at the root (*mula*) of the opposite leg, but it's not clear what he means by "root." Three of my translators illustrate the pose by showing the raised heel against the inner thigh and groin; the fourth has the raised foot across the front thigh as in Half-Lotus. We'll follow the majority and press the foot against the inner thigh.

Practice

Stand upright, feet slightly apart and parallel to each other. This is the pose we call Mountain Pose (*tadasana*). With an inhalation, shift your weight onto your right foot, keeping the inner foot pressed firmly to the floor. Look down along the midline of your torso: your sternum and navel should be directly above your right foot, so that your standing leg is slightly angled relative to the floor. Inhale again and bend your left knee;

reach down and, with your left hand, grip your left ankle. Exhale, lift your left foot up, and rest the sole against your inner right thigh. If possible, notch the heel firmly into the inner right groin, toes pointing toward the floor. Firm the left sol against the inner right thigh, and at the same time firm the outer right thigh against the sole. If you can't get the heel into the groin, simply place the foot lower down on the thigh or even the calf (but not directly against the inner knee).

Balance challenged? Don't struggle to stay upright, use a wall to brace your back, or turn your raised knee toward and push it against a wall. Or maybe you're having a hard time keeping the raised foot in place. Simply take a spare sticky mat and wedge it between the raised sole and the inner standing thigh.

Set your hands on the top rim of your pelvis. As best you can, adjust it parallel to the floor, with the two hip points parallel to the wall opposite you (assuming you're square to the walls of your practice room). Now lengthen your tailbone toward the floor, and support the lift of your chest as usual by firming your shoulder blades against your back torso. Fix your gaze on an imaginary point on the floor about 4 or 5 feet in front of you to help stabilize the pose.

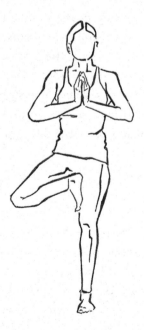

Fig. 26. Tree Pose (*vrikshasana*).

Hands and Arms

Gheranda says nothing about the hands and arms. There are two common ways to arrange them: either bring them into *anjali mudra;* or raise them vertically, holding them parallel to each other either with palms facing or with the palms pressed together, little fingers higher than the index fingers.

Traditional Benefit

None listed.

Variation

If it's possible for you to do Half-Lotus while seated on the floor, you might try the variation of Tree suggested by one of my sources. Leaning on the right foot, bend the left knee, and hug it into the belly. Keeping the knee tightly flexed, swivel the left leg; with the knee raised higher than the same-side hip, bring the outer edge of the foot into the front right hip crease. Finally, swivel the knee down and toward its mate from the left hip.

LITTLE LAMP: WHERE HAVE ALL THE STANDING POSES GONE?

Tree is the only true standing pose among the thirty-two listed by Gheranda, and none are included in the *Hatha-Yoga-Pradipika* or *Shiva-Samhita.* As a matter of fact, there are few standing poses in all of traditional Hatha Yoga. The *Hatha-Ratna-Avali* (String of Jewels on Hatha [Yoga]), a mid-seventeenth-century book, includes one among the thirty-six it describes; the *Hatha-Tatva-Kaumudi* (Moonlight on the Principles of Hatha [Yoga]), a contemporary book, lists none among its fifteen poses. So we might ask, where are all the standing poses? More than a quarter of a century ago, when I was a student at the Iyengar Institute, it was drilled into us that the two dozen or so standing poses were the foundation of the entire practice, and it was natural to imagine that it had always been so since the beginning of yoga, say, five thousand years ago.

So I guess a more accurate heading for this Little Lamp would be "Where Have All the Standing Poses Come From?" According to the *Encyclopedia of Traditional Asanas,* published by the Indian Lonavla Yoga Institute in 2006, the standing poses don't show up in yoga manuals until after about 1914 (with the one exception of the *Sacitra-Cauryayasin-Asane,* published in 1899). And where are most of the standing poses — Triangle Pose (*trikonasana*), Warrior Pose (*virabhadrasana*), Lord of the Dance Pose (*natarajasana*), Standing Forward Bend Pose (*uttanasana*), Three Steps Pose (*trivikramasana*), Hand and Foot Pose (*pada hastasana*), and even Mountain Pose (*tadasana*) — found? In a book ironically titled *Secret of Yoga (Yoga-Rahasya)* — once the book was published and distributed to the public, the secret was out of the bag — and purportedly written by the sage Nathamuni sometime in the ninth century C.E. The book was then lost for about a thousand years, until it was recovered in a vision by one of Nathamuni's descendants, a sixteen-year-old Indian by the name of Tirumular Krishnamacharya. Sound familiar? He's the éminence grise of modern yoga who, on a pilgrimage as a teenager, fell into a swoon and was visited by his distant ancestor, who dictated the contents of the lost book to him. As you might expect, not everyone believes this story about the authorship of the book, some sceptics claiming that Krishnamacharya is the book's source. Whatever the truth is, the standing poses are, without doubt, a more recent development in the evolution of the yoga asanas, certainly not more than a hundred years old.

SECTION 8: INVERSIONS

INVERSE ACTION SEAL 1

> *VIPARITA* · turned around, inverse, reverted
>
> *KARANI* · doing, making, forming
>
> *MUDRA* · seal

Inverse Action Seal (*viparita karani mudra*) more than likely started out its yoga career as something like Shoulderstand; at least that's the way all my illustrated source translations interpret it. The three main sources simply say to put the head (and hands per Gheranda) on the floor and feet in the air. But this instruction is vague enough that it could refer to a few other inversions, including Headstand. We'll take advantage of this and perform *viparita karani mudra* as both Shoulderstand and Headstand.

Henceforth, Inverse Action Seal 1 (Viparita Karani Mudra 1) will be called Shoulderstand, and Inverse Action Seal 2 (Viparita Karani Mudra 2) will be known as Headstand.

Traditional Benefit

At the least, Inverse Action Seal is said to reverse the aging process so that wrinkles and gray hair disappear. That should be enough to satisfy most of us, but wait, there's more. The successful practitioner will live virtually forever, even through the dissolution (*pralaya*) of the current universe cycle—though exactly how that works isn't explained—and presumably to be reborn in the next cycle. Needless to say, such a person has tremendous power (*siddhi*) and so is worshipped (*seva*) by the whole world (*sarva loka*).

Caution

Both Shoulderstand and (especially) Headstand require regular practice, and the supervision of an experienced teacher is highly desirable. The initial danger with Headstand is putting too much weight on the neck (the cervical vertebrae), which can cause serious neck injuries. If you are new to Headstand, don't have expert supervision, and don't feel ready to practice in the way described here (Practice 1), I recommend getting a device, available from various online sources, that will support your shoulders in an inverted position without putting any weight on your neck and head.

For Shoulderstand, it's just as imperative that you protect your neck. To this end, I highly recommend that you support your shoulders on a stack of at least three folded blankets. I'll have more to say about this in Section 10.

HEADSTAND (VIPARITA KARANI MUDRA 1)

Headstand is an exhilarating pose, especially when performed free-standing (not supported by a wall). Beginners, however, should practice against or very near a wall: if you intend to keep your heels always against the wall, then the knuckles of your clasped hands should also touch it; if you intend to balance freely for the most part and need the wall primarily for moral and only occasional physical support, then your knuckles can be a few inches away from the wall. In this section, you'll find three progressive Headstand practices. Since I can't see and correct you, the finer points that apply to your particular needs should be filled in by an experienced teacher.

Practice 1: For Beginners

Put a firm, folded blanket (made of wool or synthetic fiber, not padded) or folded sticky mat up against a clear wall (no hanging pictures, please). Kneel on the floor facing the wall. Interlace your fingers, rolling the bottom-hand pinky into the opposite hand's palm, and with your forearms on the padded floor, brace your knuckles against the wall. (Ideally,

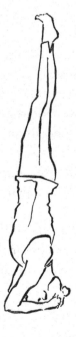

Fig. 27. Inverse Action Seal 1
(*viparita karani mudra* 1).

you should reverse the lacing of the fingers each time you practice; have the right hand higher one day, the left higher the next day, and so on.) Slide your elbows approximately shoulder-width apart, and take care that they don't slip wider while you're in the pose. Now inhale, lift your knees off the floor, and walk your feet in closer to your elbows. *Do not put your head on the floor.* You'll lift up into and come down out of the pose with your head suspended above the floor and no weight on your neck. You'll likely have to keep your knees bent as you walk your feet in.

The closer you walk your feet toward your elbows, the more likely it is that your shoulders will hunch up around your ears. Strongly draw the tops of your shoulders away from your ears, and spread your shoulder blades across your back. When your feet are as close to your elbows as possible, you're ready to take the leap of faith. The easiest way to lift off the floor is to kick up one leg at a time. This is acceptable with the head suspended, but it would be better if you tried a "bunny hop," kicking off with both feet at the same time. Just remember, whether you go up with one foot at a time or both feet together, *your head stays off the floor.* Once you're up, straighten your knees and rest your heels against the wall. It's essential that you keep your legs active during your stay in this pose, pressing through the heels and the bases of the big toes with a slight inward rotation of the thighs (so the big toes are closer than the inner heels).

Now press your inner wrists and inner elbows firmly onto the padded floor, continue lifting and spreading your shoulders wide, and lower your crown *lightly* to the floor. Keep most of your weight on your arms and shoulders. Unless you're unusually strong, you probably won't be able to stay in the pose comfortably at first for more than about 20 to 30 seconds. Don't stay to your utmost limit, when you're quaking and sweating with the effort. Reserve some strength for coming down, when you'll need to lift your head off the floor again and descend with a semblance of control. Set your sights on 20 seconds, but be prepared to abort the mission sooner if you feel your weight starting to sink onto your neck. When it's time to end the festivities, inhale; lift your head off the floor; bend your knees; and on a slow exhalation, roll down as best you can. Rest in Child's Pose.

Continue with this pose periodically over several weeks and months, depending on the regularity of your practice, gradually adding a few seconds to your stay and a bit more weight to your neck. Be reasonable with your progress, and don't be in a hurry to reach some arbitrary goal. Obviously I don't expect you to do the Original sequence every time you practice. But if you want to include Headstand in the sequence, and you're not practicing *at least* three times a week, then I recommend you stay with Practice 1, get yourself a Headstand support, or substitute Downward-Facing Dog Pose (*adho mukha shvanasana; Light on Yoga* #33). You're ready to move on to Practice 2 when you're able to hold the Practice 1 position comfortably for 3 minutes with lifted, broad shoulders and strong, active legs.

Practice 2: For Experienced Beginners

Practice 2 is pretty much the same as Practice 1, except it's now acceptable to lift up and come down from the pose with your head lightly on the floor. You might also try moving a few inches away from the wall and start to find your balance. In the best of all possible worlds, the centers of your feet will be aligned over the top of your head, so that your body makes one long line perpendicular to the floor. But it's not uncommon for the legs to be either slightly forward of or slightly behind the torso, resulting in the well-known Banana Asana. Of the two shapes, the latter is more problematic, since it puts a lot of pressure on the lower back. To correct this, lift your tailbone actively toward your heels and press your front thighs back into this resistance.

Notice, too, how your weight is distributed on your forearms. Try to bear your weight on your *inner* forearms, focusing on the inner wrists and elbows and keeping the former perpendicular to the floor. Also, distribute your weight evenly between the two forearms (so you're not tilted to one side), as well as along each forearm from the wrist to the elbow. If you find all this too difficult and the banana condition persists, then it's best to move back to and find your alignment using the wall.

When you're ready to descend, bend your knees and keep them bent as you slowly release. When you're able to hold this position comfortably for 5 minutes, maintaining your balance in a reasonably aligned position, you're ready to move along to Practice 3.

Practice 3: For Intermediates

This practice is much the same as Practice 2, except that now it's time to move away from the wall and take your chances in the middle of the room. I can assure you from my own experience that tumbling out of Headstand is no big deal; you just have to make sure you have a free-fall zone on the floor behind you (you can put some pillows there if you like — just in case) and that you have the presence of mind to release your clasped hands.

It's also time to work in earnest on lifting up with both feet leaving the floor simultaneously and coming down with both legs together. It doesn't matter right now if your knees are bent or straight, though eventually you'll want to accomplish liftoff and touchdown with straight legs.

Variation

There are literally dozens of variations of Headstand, far too many to list here. For a small sampling, see *Light on Yoga*, #74 through #86.

LITTLE LAMP: THEOS BERNARD

How long should you ultimately stay in the pose? Svatmarama suggests a daily practice of a *yama* will do the trick. How long is a *yama*? Only three hours. Of course, I'm kidding. Ten minutes is plenty for most of us. But you might wonder, is there a record of anyone actually spending three hours in Headstand? There is indeed. Here's an account by Theos Bernard, one of the earliest homegrown American yogis:

> At first it [i.e., Headstand] seemed hopeless, especially when I found out that the standard for perfection is three hours. To accomplish the goal . . . my teacher advised me to start with ten seconds for the first week and then to add thirty seconds each week until I brought the time up to fifteen minutes. This required several months. At this point I was advised to repeat the practice twice a day, which gave me a total of thirty minutes. After one month I added a midday practice period and increased the duration to twenty minutes, which gave me one hour for the day.

Thereafter I added five minutes each week until I brought up the time to a single practice period, which amounted to three hours for the day.[9]

Eventually Bernard gave up first the midday practice and then the evening one, finally combining all three into one three-hour stint.

Section 9: Abdominal Strengtheners

Peacock Pose (Mayurasana)

MAYURA · peacock

We'll divide the practice of Peacock into three parts: Practice 1 for beginners, Practice 2 for intermediates, and Practice 3 for the full pose. Have a pair of blocks or other firm supports handy for Practice 1 and a single block for Practice 2.

Practice 1: For Beginners

Set one block on one of its sides at the head of your sticky mat and a second block on one of its sides at the other end of the mat (if you only have one block, put it at the back end of the mat). Take Frog Pose exactly in the middle and facing the head of the mat. Lean forward and press your palms on the floor, fingers turned back toward your torso, thumbs pointing out to the sides; there should be an inch or so of space between the little finger sides of the hands and the outer forearms and elbows. Now bend the elbows, lean the torso forward, and walk the knees forward past the hands. Snuggle the elbows into the firm lower belly so that the chest

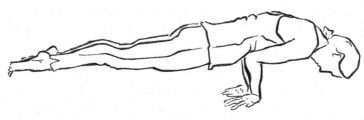

Fig. 28. Peacock Pose (*mayurasana*).

is pressed against the backs of the upper arms; with an exhalation, lay your forehead down on the block.

Reach one leg back at a time and rest the top of each foot on the second block. Stretch actively through your legs. Hold for 15 seconds, breathing as normally as possible, then bend your knees to the floor and lift out of the pose.

If your elbows tend to slip apart, try making a small loop with your yoga strap and looping it around your upper arms, just above your elbows. This should hold your arms snug when you practice the pose. But be careful: if you tip over to the side, your arms are tied together, and there's very little wiggle room.

Practice 2: For Intermediates

Practice 2 is similar to Practice 1, except there's no block for your head. After snugging your elbows into your lower belly, lay your head on the floor. When your legs are extended and you're ready to move into the pose, lift your head an inch or two off the floor and *lean your torso slightly forward,* angling your forearms relative to the floor. Hold for 15 to 20 seconds, then release your knees to the floor with an exhalation and lift out of the pose.

Practice 3: Full Pose

As described for Practice 1, snug your elbows into your lower belly. This time, though, don't lay your head on the floor as in Practice 2; instead, hold it off the floor as you reach your legs back and rest the tops of your feet on the floor. To move into the full pose, don't try to lift your feet off the floor. Instead, stretch actively back through your legs and, as in Practice 2, simply lean your torso slightly forward, angling your forearms relative to the floor (see *Light on Yoga* #127). If your legs are strong, the weight of your forward-leaning torso will lightly lever your feet off the floor. Hold for 15 to 20 seconds, then release with an exhalation.

Traditional Benefit

Both Svatmarama and Gheranda wax poetic about Peacock. Both address the pose with the honorific *shri,* which means variously "light, splendor, glory, beauty, grace; prosperity, success, auspiciousness; high rank, power, majesty." Both agree that it stokes the "fire in the belly" (*jathara agni*); destroys disease; and consumes bad food, even the most virulent poison, *kalakuta*.

LITTLE LAMP: DO YOGA, LIVE FOREVER

There are a few exaggerated or unsubstantiated claims in our modern yoga books about the benefits of the various asanas. But nothing in them matches the wild claims made by the traditional books about the benefits of asanas and mudras. "Conquer death" is probably at the top of the list, closely followed by "conquer disease," and—a personal favorite of mine—"reverse the aging process." These are all relatively benign allegations, but one seems particularly dangerous. Do Peacock, it says, and you can drink and easily digest "lethal poison," which is how one of my sources renders *kalakuta*, literally "black substance." Now *kalakuta* isn't just any lethal poison, it's the most lethal substance ever produced. To save the world from its deadly effects, Shiva drank the stuff, which then turned his throat blue, earning him the nickname *nila kantha* (Blue Throat).

Caution

Obviously if you have any problems with either or both of your wrists, or if you're pregnant, then you should avoid this pose.

Variation

Peacock doesn't lack for variations. You can twist the legs to one side and rest them on the back of the bent arm. This is equivalent to Iyengar's Two-Legs Koundinya's Pose (*dvi pada koundinyasana; Light on Yoga* #158; Koundinya being an obscure Vedic sage). You can perform the pose with the legs in Lotus. Iyengar calls this Lotus-Peacock Pose (*padma mayurasana; Light on Yoga* # 128). You can also perform the pose with one leg stretched behind the torso and one leg stretched out to the side, with the inner thigh resting on the back of the same-side upper arm; Iyengar calls this One-Leg Koundinya's Pose II (*eka pada koundinyasana; Light on Yoga* #160). Finally, you can twist one leg to rest on the back of the opposite-side arm and stretch the second leg out behind the torso, which Iyengar calls One-Leg Koundinya's Pose I (*eka pada koundinyasana; Light on Yoga* #159).

VAJROLI SEAL (VAJROLI MUDRA)

VAJROLI · untranslated here

Vajroli Seal provides us with an interesting contrast between Svatmarama's practice and Gheranda's. By the end of the seventeenth century, Vajroli is a tame asana-like exercise similar to what we call Full Boat Pose (*paripurna navasana*), which is how we'll treat it in this sequence. But in the earlier *Hatha-Yoga-Pradipika*, Vajroli is a horse of an entirely different color. I suspect it's a remnant of an old Tantric practice, assimilated by Hatha Yoga, in which male and female practitioners engage in ritual intercourse.

We'll look more closely at Svatmarama's Vajroli in this section's Little Lamp. For now, let's move along to Gheranda's less controversial, solo version. The heading for this section is "Abdominal Strengtheners." Ideally, this exercise strengthens the *deep* abdominal, or psoas, muscles, which run from the lower spine across the back of the pelvis, over the pubis, and insert into the inner thighbones. These are truly "core" muscles, integrating the spine, pelvis, and legs, and serve primarily as hip flexors (they lift and flex the hip joints); though, of course, when the legs are fixed, they pull the torso into a forward bend. The psoas muscles

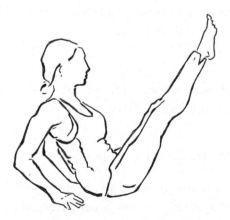

Fig. 29. Vajroli Seal
(Vajroli *mudra*).

are also closely related to what I call the "roots" of the diaphragm, formally known as the crura (*crus* in singular form). These comprise a pair of long, skinny muscles reaching down like pigtails from the back of the diaphragm and attaching to the lower (lumbar) spine. Thus, the psoas muscles affect not only movement and posture but breathing as well. The superficial abdominal muscles (or rectus abdominis muscles), which run from the lower ribs down to the pubis, will be firmed by this practice but shouldn't harden and mound up.

Practice

Sit in Staff Pose. Lean your torso back slightly and press your hands to the floor just behind your pelvis, with the fingers pointing forward. Bend your knees and set your feet on the floor. Inhale, exhale, and raise your feet a few inches off the floor, so your thighs and torso form an approximate right angle. Hold for a few breaths. If you can go further, maintaining the angle between torso and thighs, bend your knees and raise your forelegs until they're parallel to the floor. Hold for a few more breaths. Finally, if possible, straighten your knees and press actively through your heels. If you find it difficult to hold your knees straight, wrap a strap around the soles and hold the ends firmly in your hands, pushing through your heels. If and when you feel steady, let go of the strap, press your hands back on the floor, and hold the position for as long as possible.

Your front torso may tend to sag a bit, so firm your shoulder blades against your back torso and lift the top of your sternum. Hold for 15 to 30 seconds, then bend your knees and release your feet to the floor. You may repeat this exercise two or three times if you like.

Traditional Benefit

According to Gheranda, Vajroli brings about a "life that lasts a long time" (*cira jiva*) and awakens *shakti*, another name for *kundalini*.

Little Lamp: Svatmarama's Vajroli Seal

Svatmarama's Vajroli is covered in nine verses in his chapter on mudras. Without going into detail, the practice involves ritual intercourse, the purpose of which is the preservation and transformation of sexual fluids, both male and female. David Gordon White comments,

> The male practitioner, having ejaculated into his female partner, withdraws his own semen, now catalyzed through its interaction with her sexual essence . . . back into his own body. In so doing, he also draws back into himself, along with his own refined seed, a certain quantity of that female essence which may in turn serve to catalyze yogic processes (the raising of the kundalini, etc.) by which his semen becomes transmuted into nectar.[10]

In the predominantly sexually conservative culture of modern yoga, this Vajroli has created, as you might expect, varying degrees of discomfort for our translators. The offending verses have basically been treated in five different ways.

1. Ignore the verses or condemn them as an aberration, as in this example:

> The following slokas . . . are practices that aim at reversing the flow of the semen virile in coito. The purpose of such practices is clear: to enjoy all the benefits of yoga without sacrificing any of the worldly pleasures.
>
> In leaving out these passages, we merely bypass the description of a few obscure and repugnant practices that are followed only by yogis who lack the will power to reach their goal otherwise. In these . . . slokas, we encounter a yoga that has nothing but its name in common with the yoga of a Patanjali or a Ramakrishna.[11]

2. Mistranslate the verses.

3. Translate the verses but spin the interpretation. Some authors claim that the obvious interpretation, that the practice involves a form of intercourse, is mistaken and that only ignorant people would think that way; in actuality, the practice represents some nonphysical process.

4. Translate the verses but claim that only qualified married couples should try it.

5. Translate the verses and revel in them, as shown in this example:

The auspicious practice of vajroli not only brings about the vast material pleasure but as well as [sic] immortality to man. (*Hatha-Tatva-Kaumudi* 16.16)

Here we see how, even 350 years ago, traditional yoga was changed to make it more acceptable to the dominant culture.

SECTION 10: INVERSION 2

SHOULDERSTAND, INVERSE ACTION SEAL (VIPARITA KARANI MUDRA 2)

Whenever I see students performing Shoulderstand with their shoulders flat on the floor, I get a sympathetic ache in my neck. I'm aware that some schools of modern Hatha Yoga eschew the use of props, and that's generally okay—though not, in my humble opinion, always the best way to go about the work. When it comes to Shoulderstand, however, I must insist that the shoulders be lifted off the floor on a blanket support, somewhere between 2 and 6 inches thick.

If you're not accustomed to using a blanket support, you might well be asking yourself, why? Find a mirror and stand sideways to it. Lift your chest and lower your chin toward your sternum; don't force it, just bow your head. Without moving too much, try to peek at yourself in the mirror. Draw an imaginary line along the back torso; if you're standing more or less upright, it should be about perpendicular to the floor. Now draw another line along the back of your neck from the base of your skull until it intersects the back torso line. (This is a lot like high school geometry, isn't it?) Estimate the degree of angle formed by the two lines. It's unlikely that they'll form a right angle (that is, 90 degrees); more probably, the angle will be somewhat greater than 90 degrees.

If you have a copy of *Light on Yoga*, look at plate #234 (if you don't have a copy, you'll just have to trust me on this one). There's Mr. Iyengar in Shoulderstand with his shoulders flat on the floor. Again, draw the two lines along the back torso and back neck. What's the angle? About as close to 90 degrees as you can get. Are you starting to catch the drift of this long-winded explanation? If you do a flat-on-the-floor Shoulderstand, in order to get your torso vertical, your neck has to bend to 90 degrees. Most of us can't do that comfortably, as you experienced with the mirror experiment. So as a consequence, one of two things will happen:

1. You won't be able to get your torso vertical, in which case you'll be forced to hold yourself up muscularly instead of being lightly balanced on the tops of your shoulders (yes, that's why they call it *Shoulder*stand). This, in turn, will result in a good deal of struggle and unpleasantness.

2. You'll force your torso to the vertical, and either right away or eventually, you'll strain your neck, possibly even flattening the natural cervical curve.

Convinced?

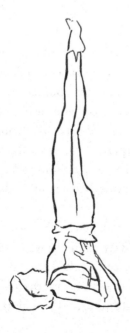

Fig. 30. Inverse Action Seal 2 (*viparita karani mudra* 2).

Preliminary

Even among blanket advocates, there's some controversy about how many blankets to use. As a rule of thumb, I have beginning Shoulder-standers use a minimum of three blankets. It's rare for a student to need fewer but common to need more. At any rate, fold your blankets into rectangles of approximately 2 feet by 3 feet. Notice that of the two long edges, one is firmly folded and the other is open; stack the long, firm edges atop each other. This is your Shoulderstand support.

It's best to time yourself while in this pose. Set a watch on the floor (with its face upside down) where you can see it.

LITTLE LAMP: LYING ON THE BLANKET SUPPORT

When lying on the support, your head should be on the floor, your shoulders on the long, firm side and a few inches in from the edge of the blankets. Once you're in this position, *be sure not to turn your head.* Continue to keep your head in a neutral position, looking straight up.

Practice 1: For Beginners

Beginners should set the long, open edges of their blankets 6 inches to a foot away from an open wall. Lie down on the support, and with bent knees, put your feet on the wall. Inhale and, pressing your feet against the wall, lift your back torso away from the floor. Keep your feet on the wall for a while longer, and try to bring your pelvis directly over your shoulders so that your torso and thighs are perpendicular to the floor. Bend your elbows and bring your hands, palms flat, to your midback, pressing firmly with the ring and little fingers. If your elbows tend to slip apart, support them on a rolled-up sticky mat.

If this is your first time trying Shoulderstand, or if you're relatively new to the practice, inhale and take one foot away from the wall, straighten the knee, and press through the heel to the ceiling. Hold for 10 seconds, then put that foot back on the wall and do the same with the second leg. If you feel ready, take both feet off the wall and press through the heels.

Stay for 30 seconds. Bend your knees, return your feet to the wall, and come down on an exhalation. I know this seems like a short stay, but it's best to start out modestly and add 10 to 15 seconds a week to your stay until you reach 3 minutes.

If you have more experience with this pose, then you can take both feet off the wall together and hold initially for a minute or so. Shoulderstand and Headstand are, sorry to say, everyday poses, and if you're unable or unwilling to make a strong commitment to practicing them a *minimum* of four to six times each week, then it's best to leave them (at least Headstand) out of your sequence. When you reach the end of your stay, exhale your feet back to the wall and lower your torso to the floor. The proximal goal is to stay comfortably for 3 minutes, then to increase to 5 minutes. When you've reached the latter stage and are ready to go further, it's time to get instruction from a living teacher.

Practice 2: For Intermediates

Since I assume intermediates already have a Shoulderstand practice, I won't say too much about it, because the details are endless. Let me mention two points I think are important. Throughout your stay in the pose, keep your legs firm and your heels pressing toward the ceiling. I see way too many students practice this pose with floppy legs, which puts too much weight on the shoulders and neck. Also, press your outer elbows to the support, and try to lift the base of your neck (at the seventh cervical vertebra) off the floor. This, again, will help take pressure off the neck.

Traditional Benefit

Remember that Shoulderstand was originally a mudra. For Gheranda, doing this practice regularly "annihilates, destroys" (*nasha*) old age (*jara*) and death (*mrita*), and it makes the practitioner an adept (*siddha*) who will survive even the next dissolution of the universe (*pralaya*)—which I understand is due in 2012 (and I hope you're reading this in 2013). Svatmarama says the practitioner will win out over death, but only if the pose is practiced for 3 hours daily (*yama matra,* "measure of a *yama,*" an eighth of a day or 3 hours).

LITTLE LAMP: HEELS OVER HEAD

Why do we want to invert ourselves anyway? Modern books talk about the many health benefits of an inverted position but don't say much about the original purpose. And no wonder; the story seems entirely fantastic to our modern sensibility. It involves a mysterious, subtle fluid my sources call "deathless" (*amrita*), though it's also known by other exotic names like "juice" (*soma*), "nectar" (*sudha*, literally "good drink," or *piyusha*), and "immortal liquor" (*amara varuna*). This nectar is said to drip from the "moon" (*shasha*), a subtle center located either at the back of the throat or the base of the brain. In the upright position in which nonyogis spend their lives, this fluid falls into the "sun" (*surya*), in the solar plexis or navel, where it's burned up and wasted. The nonyogi thus ages and expires after a normal life span. But in the yogi's upside-down position, the nectar is preserved in the head (helped out by the Net-Bearing–like position of the neck and head), where she can drink it to her heart's content. As a result, as the name of the fluid suggests, the yogi remains youthful-looking and lives far beyond a human's normally allotted time on earth. In fact, Anonymous/Gheranda and Anonymous/Shiva claim the yogi doesn't even die when the whole universe comes to an end (*pralaya*).

But even more, turning ourselves upside down inverts our world. This is what Hatha Yoga traditionally was meant to do, to reverse the "natural order" of the world. So we find exercises to open what's blocked (for example, *sushumna nadi*) and block what's open (such as the throat or anus); to lift what wants to go down (for example, *apana vayu*) and push down what wants to go up (such as *prana vayu*); and to stop what wants to move back and forth (which means to stop the pendulum-like movement of time and live in the unmoving present).

SECTION 11: PERFECTED FAMILY

The Perfected Family, as I'm calling it, is named after the most notable of its five members, the Perfected Pose (*siddhasana*). To a casual observer,

Name	Feet	Body	Other
Auspicious (*svastika*)	Wedged in opposite bent-leg crease	Sitting straight	
Cowherd (*goraksha*)	On opposite bent-leg crease, soles visible	Head in *jalandhara bandha* Eyes in *nasa agra drishti*	
Secret (*gupta*)	Hidden in opposite bent-leg crease, sitting on heel		
Freedom (*mukta*)	Ankles crossed	Sitting straight	Sitting for listening to *nada* (see chapter 7)
Perfected (*siddha*)	One heel pressing perineum, the other heel pressing the penis	Head in *jalandhara bandha* Eyes in *bhru madhya drishti*	Sense organs restrained (*samyama*)

the members might seem like quintuplets, so close are they to one another in outward appearance. But the differences between them, though subtle, are significant, and sequenced in a certain way (though not in the haphazard order listed by Gheranda), they comprise a more or less logical progression.

Preliminary: Alternate Crossing

For all five poses, begin by sitting in Staff Pose. No matter which pose or poses you may be practicing, be sure to alternate the cross of the legs day by day; don't get into the habit of crossing them the same way all the time. My rule of thumb is right leg higher on even-numbered days and left leg higher on odd-numbered days during even-numbered years; conversely, left leg higher on even-numbered days and right leg higher on odd-numbered days in odd-numbered years. (I know this seems overly technical, but I do this year-by-year reversal because there are seven more odd-numbered than even-numbered days in a year.)

Caution

If you have a groin or knee injury, do your sitting practice in Easy Pose (*sukhasana*), with the shins crossed, the feet positioned under the opposite-side knees, and the knees supported on blocks or folded blankets if necessary.

AUSPICIOUS POSE (SVASTIKASANA)

> SVASTIKA · fortunate, auspicious (from *su*, "well, good,"
> and *asti*, "being," meaning "all is well")

Since Easy Pose (*sukhasana*) isn't included in this book, we'll use Auspicious (see fig. 10, page 117) as the basic sitting posture.

Practice

From Staff, bend both knees and set your feet on the floor. Lay your left leg off to the side and down on the floor; slide the heel close to but not right against the left sitting bone. Lift your right foot and wiggle the outer edge (little-toe side) into the crease between the left thigh and calf. Lay the right leg on the floor, or support the knee on a block if needed. Draw the heels up to the perineum, and try to wiggle the inner edge (big-toe side) of the left foot into the crease between the right thigh and calf. Sit with a "straight body" (*riju kaya*).

Traditional Benefit

None are listed in either the *Hatha-Yoga-Pradipika* or the *Gheranda-Samhita*. The *Hatha-Tatva-Kaumudi* (7.45–46) and the *Shiva-Samhita* (3.113–115), however, do list benefits. The former tells us that Auspicious cures fatigue and anxiety and confers mental peace and happiness (*shanti*). Shiva recommends this "seat" for *pranayama*, saying that sitting in Auspicious will help the yogi master the "wind" (*vayu*), or *prana*. He adds that this pose destroys "all suffering" (*sarva duhkha*).

COWHERD OR GORAKSHA'S POSE (GORAKSHASANA)

> *GO* · cow
>
> *RAKSHA* · guard, watcher, keeper; a tutelary divinity

This pose is dedicated to Goraksha, whose fame as a Hatha yogin is second only to that of Matsyendra. Traditional Cowherd looks nothing like its modern Iyengar incarnation (see *Light on Yoga* #54), a sort of balance-on-your-knees-in-Lotus (and hope for the best) exercise. Instead, traditional Cowherd builds on Auspicious by adding a bond (*bandha*) and a gaze (*drishti*).

Practice

Arrange your feet similarly to Auspicious, but don't snug the edges of the feet into the thigh-calf creases. Instead, rest the feet on the opposite thigh-calf crease with the soles "visible" (*vyakta*). Cover the upper heel with your stacked hands, with the back of one resting in the palm of the other. Perform Net-Bearing Bond and Tip-of-the-Nose Gaze (*nasa agra drishti*).

Traditional Benefit

Cowherd brings unspecified success (*siddha*; which is explained more fully at Perfected Pose).

LITTLE LAMP: GORAKSHA

Goraksha is a semilegendary figure who is said to have lived anywhere from the ninth to the twelfth centuries. He's thought by many to be the founder of Hatha Yoga and the order of "split-ear" (*kanphata*) yogis, so called because their initiation ceremony involves piercing the novice's ear cartilage and inserting a large earring. This ceremony has largely been dropped from modern yoga classes.

Secret Pose (Guptasana)

GUPTA · protected, hidden, secret

In this pose, the feet are hidden, or "kept secret," below the pelvis.

Practice

From Auspicious, slide the feet completely between the opposite leg's thigh-calf crease, then sit on the heels.

Traditional Benefit

None listed.

Little Lamp: Listen, Do You Want to Know a Secret? (Do You Promise Not to Tell?)

Many centuries ago, the teachings of yoga were kept in the strictest secrecy, given to only a select group of students who had proved to the teacher their dedication to the practice beyond a shadow of a doubt. Why the secrecy? Heinrich Zimmer explains,

> Wisdom, in the Orient, no matter what its kind, is to be guarded jealously and communicated sparingly, and then only to one capable of becoming its perfect receptacle, for besides representing a certain skill, every department of learning carries with it a power that can amount almost to magic, a power to bring to pass what without it would seem a miracle. Teaching not intended to communicate such power is simply of no consequence, and the communication to one unfit to wield the power properly would be disastrous. Furthermore, the possession of the wisdom and its special potencies was in ancient times regarded as one of the most valuable portions of the family heritage. Like a treasure, it was handed down with all care, according to the patrilineal order of descent. Charms, spells, the techniques of the various crafts and professions, and, finally, philosophy itself originally were communicated only in this way.[12]

Nowadays of course, yoga is broadcast far and wide to every big city and backwater in the world. For a few dollars, we can buy or find free online books—like the *Rigveda* or any of the Upanishads—that were once considered more precious than Bill Gates's bank account.

We might ask why has this happened, who let the yoga cat out of the bag? One theory I have is called the Hand-Me-Down Theory. It proposes that the once-secret practices have become obsolete for traditional yogis, that they've found more effective methods—which of course they're holding in the strictest secrecy—and have simply passed along their worn-out spiritual "rags" to their little-brother masses.

When I explained this to a friend, she suggested—strongly—that the theory was much too cynical. So to placate her, I came up with another called the Guinea Pig Theory. It proposes that the centuries of secrecy were necessary while the old yogis tested the practices on themselves, so they could fine-tune them without interference and make sure they were safe for the rest of us before going public. I later found some justification for this theory from Herr Zimmer:

> In ninety days [Nagarjuna] studied and mastered the whole of the Buddhist Pali canon. Then he proceeded northward, in quest of further knowledge, until he came to the Himalayas, where a monk of immense age committed to him the Mahayana sutras; after which a serpent king (*nagaraja*) disclosed an authentic commentary on those pages. All these sacred writings had been preserved in secret—so the story goes—for centuries. They were, in fact, authentic revelations of the doctrine, which the Buddha himself had regarded as too profound for his contemporaries and had therefore put into the keeping of competent guardians. Mankind had required literally hundreds of years of preliminary training (the training of the Hinayana) in preparation for this higher law. But now that the world was ready, Nagarjuna was permitted to spread the final Buddhist teaching of The Great Ferryboat throughout the land of India.[13]

It's still an interesting exercise to keep some of your yoga knowledge secret from others, to preserve in a small way the original playful charm and specialness of the practice. As Johan Huizinga remarks,

The exceptional and special position of play is most tellingly illustrated by the fact that it loves to surround itself with an air of
secrecy. Even in early childhood the charm of play is enhanced
by making a secret out of it. This is for *us*, not for the others.
What the others do outside is no concern of ours at the moment.
Inside the circle of the game the laws and customs of ordinary
life no longer count. We are different and do things differently.[14]

Or to paraphrase Svatmarama (*Hatha-Yoga-Pradipika* 1.11), yoga wisdom
should be "top secret" (*param gopya*) by the yogi who wants to succeed
(*siddhi*). This wisdom is "powerful" (*virya*) when held secret and "un-
powerful" (*nirvirya*) when public or visible (*prakasha*).

FREEDOM POSE (MUKTASANA)

MUKTA · loosened, set free, relaxed, open; liberated,
   delivered, emancipated (especially from sin or worldly
   existence); fallen or dropped down (as fruit); abandoned,
   sent forth, left free (as a road), gone, vanished; the spirit
   released from corporeal existence

This pose can also be called Liberated Pose. Do you want to be liberated
in the traditional meaning of the word? I imagine that many serious yoga
students have pondered this question, and many of them have answered
in the affirmative. All I can say is, be careful what you ask for. Have you
considered the possibility that liberation means a radical change in your
identity, not to mention your life?

The picture Gheranda draws of the moment of liberation is both
appealing and troublesome. We will realize the awesome oneness of
all life—that the creatures of the earth (*bhucara*) and air (*kha*), all the
plants, all water or fluid (*vari*), and the mountains (*parvati*) are Brahman, and Brahman is the self (*atman*). But then he writes that the self
is equivalent to consciousness (*chaitanya*), which upon liberation is
"split, broken" (*bhinna*) apart from the body, which seems to contradict
his previous statement about affirming the oneness of life. But the yogi's
self is not only separated from his body; in liberation, he's also emotion-

ally separated from his children (*putra*), wife (*dara*), friends, and all of life around him. It seems to me — and of course, I'm not liberated — the insight that all is Brahman, including my own self, would instill in me an immense appreciation for and deep love of life, even including my daughter when she refuses to clean up her room.

Svatmarama's description is no more alluring. After all our hard work to purify and "bake" the body to make it a suitable vehicle for the goddess, in the end it becomes like a piece of "wood" (*kashtha*) and the yogi is "dead" to the world — not sensing, not even breathing. This is surely an aspect of traditional Hatha Yoga that has no place in its modern incarnation. Surely liberation is inclusive of all life, so we feel a close kinship to all living things and a powerful urge to share our insight with anyone who expresses an interest (and even a few who don't).

Practice

Cross your ankles and sit on the top heel. Keep your body (*kaya*), head (*shira*), and neck (*griva*) straight.

Traditional Benefit

Freedom Pose brings unspecified success (*siddha*; explained at Perfected Pose).

PERFECTED POSE (SIDDHASANA)

SIDDHA · accomplished, fulfilled, thoroughly skilled or versed in; perfected, beatified; endowed with supernatural faculties, sacred, holy, divine; one who has attained the highest object

Svatmarama devotes one or two verses to twelve of his fifteen asanas. Of the remaining three poses, three verses go to Lion, six to Lotus, and ten to Perfected. Why the great disparity? Svatmarama rates Perfected as the best and most comfortable of all the asanas, a high honor indeed when you consider there are 8.4 million and no other asana can compare. He puts it in the Yoga Hall of Fame along with the other practices that signify a "perfected" practitioner: *kevala kumbhaka* (see chapter 7);

khechari mudra (see chapter 6); and *laya yoga,* the yoga of "dissolution" (that is, the limited self).

Anonymous/Shiva also rates Perfected very highly, though not as highly as Svatmarama. Anonymous/Gheranda is far less impressed with the pose; he gives it one measly verse copied almost word for word from Svatmarama.

Practice

Svatmarama gives two versions for the feet and legs in this practice. It seems that the majority of practitioners do the pose with one heel pressed against the perineum and the other foot on the penis. Then he cites an unnamed source who performs the pose with the left ankle pressing above the penis and the right ankle above the left heel.

I've made a number of different suggestions of what to do with your hands in sitting poses throughout this book. The easiest is to either lay your hands in your lap, palms up, one hand stacked in the other, or lay your hands on your knees. With you hands on your knees you have two choices: palms up tends to help open the chest, and palms down tends to help release the shoulders. Try them both out to see which one suits you best.

While some call this *siddha,* he continues, others call it Diamond Pose, Freedom Pose, or Secret Pose. It appears from this that, even in Svatmarama's time, not all the teachers agreed on the name and arrangement of many of the poses.

Presumably, both versions include Svatmarama's further instructions to perform Net-Bearing Bond and *bhru madhya drishti,* to restrain

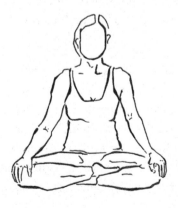

Fig. 31. Perfected Pose
(*siddhasana*).

(*samyama*) the senses, and to sit motionless (*sthira*). Shiva tells us that Perfected is the pose that should be used regularly as a seat for *pranayama*.

Traditional Benefit

Svatmarama remarks (and Gheranda copies) that *siddha* breaks open the door (*kapata*) to liberation (*moksha*), an excellent reason this pose ranks as number one. It also purifies the (seventy-two thousand) *nadis*, though exactly how it does this isn't mentioned.

Shiva, too, is enthusiastic about Perfected. He notes that practicing the pose grants "perfection" to the practitioner, although he also says that the same happens merely by reflecting (*dhyana*) on it. No wonder he calls it the greatest pose on earth (*bhuvana*) that helps us reach the ultimate (*para*).

LITTLE LAMP: THE MEANING
OF THE SANSKRIT *SIDDHA*

I haven't counted all the words in the *Hatha-Yoga-Pradipika*, but I'll bet that one of the more common is *siddha*. By my informal tally, it's used forty-four times and has various meanings. The word is rooted in the verb *sidh*, "to succeed." It variously means one who is

- "accomplished, fulfilled," and has "gained" the highest object and is thoroughly "skilled or versed" in yoga, and so is "perfected";
- endowed with supernatural faculties (*sindhi*), and so is "effective, powerful, miraculous";
- "sacred, illustrious"; or
- "healed" or "cured," presumably both physically and spiritually.

SECTION 12: RELAXATION

CORPSE POSE (SHAVASANA)

> SHAVA · corpse (from *shav*, "to go, approach"; "to alter, change, transform")

Corpse is also known as *mrita asana*, "Death Pose" (see *Gheranda-Samhita* 2.4). "Corpse" and "Death" might seem like odd names for a yoga pose. It's not likely in this day and age that anyone selling yoga products or services would name them after a dead body. And attitudes haven't changed that much since Svatmarama's time; 650 years ago, the average Indian was no less repelled by a corpse than we are today. There must be at least a dozen other Sanskrit words that could have represented this pose just as effectively, getting across the idea to lie very still. Of course, we first have to recognize that the men who labeled these poses weren't your average Indians, but rather voluntary pariahs who weren't concerned with the usual social niceties. It could be that the term *corpse* was chosen at least partially for its shock value, directed at the yogis themselves since these practices weren't generally public knowledge. We know for sure that some schools of Hatha encouraged its members to frequent graveyards and to meditate there on the transience of life while perched on a corpse no less—quite literally a *shavasana*, "corpse seat." Death, too, had a different meaning for these men; it stood not for the much-feared end of worldly life, but for the death of their limited ego identity and their final release from existential suffering.

LITTLE LAMP: SHAVA SADHANA

Want to practice historically authentic Hatha Yoga? Well, here's how the real *shavasana* is performed. John Woodroffe says,

> In *Shava sadhana* the *sadhaka* (literally, "skillful person") sits astride on the back of a corpse (heading north), on which he draws a *yantra* [cosmic diagram] and then does *japa* [repetition] of *mantra* with *shodha nyasa* ["purifying touch"] and *puja*

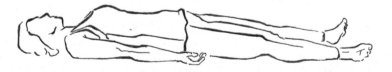

Fig. 32. Corpse Pose (*shavasana*).

["worship"] on its head. A corpse is selected as being a pure form of organized matter, since the *devata* [deity] which is invoked into it is *maha vidya* ["great wisdom"] whose *svarupa* ["true form"] is *nirguna brahman* ["qualityless brahman"], and by such invocation becomes *saguna* ["with quality"]. The corpse is free from sin or desire. The only *vayu* in it is the *dhanam jaya* [conquest of the prize], "which leaves not even a corpse." The *devata* materializes by means of the corpse. There is a possession of it—that is, entry of the *devata* into the dead body. At the conclusion of a successful rite, it is said that the head of the corpse turns round, and facing the *sadhaka*, speaks, bidding him name his boon, which may be spiritual or worldly advancement as he wishes. This is part of *nila* ["dark blue"] *sadhana* done by the hero (*vira*) for it and *shavasana* are attended by many terrors.[15]

And don't forget to face north.

Corpse ostensibly tells us what to do physically in the pose—pretend we're dead—but I believe it also tells us what to do psychically. For the yogis, *shava* is a not-so-subtle reference to Shiva, the patron saint of Hatha. It's a well-known teaching that Shiva without his *i* (which stands for Sanskrit *iccha*, "will, desire, inclination") is *shava* (in Sanskrit, remove the *i* from Shiva, and it's automatically replaced with an *a*). Shiva-as-*shava* represents the passive, "will-less" witnessing agent (*sakshin*, "eye witness"); the inactive, universal consciousness. And what is he witnessing? His spouse and inseparable complement, Shakti ("power, ability, energy, capability"), the active, willful force or creative power of the universe. In *shava*, then, we consciously assume the role of the Witness—which is "choiceless awareness" according to Jiddu Krishnamurti—with no expectation or judgment, simply looking at what is.

We may look physically dead to an uninformed observer because we're so completely unmoving, but it's not because we're dead to the world; rather, we're unqualifiedly absorbed in the play of our own inner processes, whether it be our breath or the "fluctuations" (*vritti*) of our mind's contents. Paradoxically in Corpse, our inner world is in a condition of heightened "aliveness" that feeds itself because it is what we long for more than anything else: the more closely and consistently we watch, the more alive we become; the more alive we become, the more closely and consistently we can watch.

I won't go into the meaning of the graveyard in traditional Hatha Yoga practice, except to say that for the yogi it represents not a place of horror and disgust, but an arena of self-transformation, a place where the false concept of self-limitation is symbolically "laid to rest." The "corpse" (*shava*) is actually the lord of the graveyard, who in another role is Shiva, the patron saint of Hatha Yoga. Shiva is Shava, and Shiva ("in whom all things lie") is forever joined to his spouse, Shakti, the power holder and the "power" (*shak*, "to be able"). Here Shiva is the passive Witness to his consort's world play (*lila*). In Corpse Pose, the stillness of the physical body imitates a corpse, but not because it's "dead." Rather, so enthralled is the God by the Goddess's dance, that he's motionless in rapt attention, all the better to focus his consciousness entirely on the beauty and joy of her creation. The other essential element is called "presence" in English, from the root *esse*, "to be," or *sat* in Sanskrit, "being or being present." While the body may look corpselike, consciousness (*chitta*) is experiencing life to the fullest, watching itself play in the world mirror it self-creates. This leads to *ananda*, "pure happiness," the ultimate goal of yoga.

There are three essential elements of a successful Corpse:

1. Balance (from *bilancia,* which means "having two scale pans")
2. Stillness (from *stha,* which means "to stand")
3. Presence (from *es,* which means "to be")

I'll explain what I mean by these qualities as we work on the pose. You might want a folded blanket to pillow your head, another blanket to cover yourself if your practice room isn't heated, and a eye bag to cover your eyes. Ready to start?

Practice

The first element of Corpse is *balance,* which applies to the physical body. Imagine that the two sides of your body are like the pans of an old-fashioned scale, your midline (a line drawn exactly down the middle of your body that divides it perfectly in half) is the fulcrum on which the pans' balance arm swings. Lie on your back and rock gently side to side a bit, trying to balance the weight of the two sides of your torso on the floor so the "scale pans" are level with each other.

Arrange your limbs and head evenly relative to the midline. Your heels, ideally only a few inches apart, should each rest on the same spot, so your turned-out feet are angled evenly to an imaginary line drawn midway between them perpendicular to the floor. Your arms should each be angled at about 45 degrees relative to the sides of your torso, with each hand resting on the same knuckle, preferably that of the index finger. Finally, your head should be neutral, with your ears equidistant from your shoulders and your eyes equidistant from the ceiling.

The second element, *stillness*, has both a detailed and a more general application. In regard to the former, pay especial attention to your tongue, eyes, and the skin at the bridge of your nose. Your tongue should ideally rest on the floor of your mouth, spreading outward from its own midline and releasing from its tip along its sides deep into the throat. Your eyes should sink back in their sockets and turn down. You might find it challenging at first to keep your eyes still; even though your lids are closed, your eyes habitually want to move around as if looking at the room. So you'll have to check back periodically and, if need be, inhibit their movement.

The area between your eyebrows at the bridge of your nose is called the glabella, the "hairless" spot. This skin is attached to the forehead muscle (the frontalis) underneath, which in turn has a stimulating or quieting effect on the brain, depending on whether it's tense or relaxed. Bring awareness to the quality of this skin. Imagine it softening and seeming to melt away from the nose bridge to either side toward the temples.

The stilling of the eyes and softening of the skin both have a quieting effect on the brain, which Iyengar singles out as the most difficult organ to adjust. Can you imagine your brain cradled inside your skull? If you can, let it first sink to the back of the skull, then let it shrink to a small ball. It's especially important for the brain to stay back and remain small during your inhalations, which tend to inflate and stimulate the brain. Once all this is in place, resolve to remain as physically still and corpselike as possible for however long you stay in the pose.

Finally, the third element of the pose is *presence*. We often have a difficult time staying present or awake in this pose, particularly in the late
afternoon or evening when we're tired and tend to drift off to sleep or
into a dreamlike reverie. Strengthening presence is like strengthening a
muscle, it initially requires some will power not to accede to the allure
of mind, to determinedly bring your awareness back to the present each
time you lose the thread.

TURN OUT THE LIGHT

I've taught this sequence for many years at my home base in Oakland,
California, and around the country. There's something about it, I'm told,
that is subtly transformative, at least temporarily. Obviously you won't
want to practice the Original asana sequence every day, though it might
be worthwhile to take it on daily at some point in the future for a week or
two straight. I try to practice it about once or twice a month or anytime I
just don't feel like trying to figure out what to do. As I said, the sequence
isn't carved in stone; it's not trademarked; and you won't be sued if, as
a teacher, you present it to your class and are not "certified" to do so —
mostly because there is no certification. I do ask that if you teach it, you
present it just the way it is in this chapter three or four times before you
decide to improve on my many flaws. It would be good if you first had
a feel for the sequence before you changed it in any way. And if you do
change it, try to keep the number of poses at thirty-two. Let's do that as
an acknowledgment of Gheranda and all his traditional colleagues.

6

SEALS AND BONDS: *MUDRAS* AND *BANDHAS*

MUDRA • a seal or any instrument used for
sealing or stamping, seal ring, signet ring; the stamp or
impression made by a seal; any stamp, print, mark, or
impression; image, sign, badge, token (especially a
token or mark of divine attributes impressed on
the body); shutting, closing (as of the eyes or
lips); particular positions or intertwinings
of the fingers

BANDHA • binding, tying; bond, tie, chain, fetter;
damming up (e.g., a river); capture, arrest; imprisonment,
custody; putting together, uniting, contracting, combining,
forming, producing; any configuration or position of
the body (especially of the hands and feet); fixing,
directing (mind, eyes, etc.)

A *MUDRA IS A* "SEAL," an English word that more or less accurately
relays by itself the Sanskrit meaning. "Seal" can be either a noun or a
verb. As the former, my dictionary defines it as an instrument, such as
a die or signet ring, with a "raised or incised emblem used to stamp an
impression on a receptive substance such as wax or lead." As the latter,
it means "to close with or as if with a seal." In practical terms, a mudra
physically "seals" up the body in some way, preventing a "leak" of consciousness or *pranic* energy.

Generally there are three categories of seals. Perhaps the most familiar are the hand (*hasta*) seals, of which *jnana mudra* or the pressed-together-palms gesture called *anjali mudra* may be the best known. Hand seals aren't mentioned by our revered teachers.

LITTLE LAMP: HAND SEALS (*HASTA MUDRAS*)

A seal often has, along with its practical application, a symbolic interpretation; its shape is said to "stamp" a certain meaning on the practitioner's body. Take, for example, the well-known hand gesture called the Wisdom Seal (*jnana mudra*), in which the tips of the thumb and index finger are pressed together, forming a circle, while the remaining three fingers are pressed together side by side and extended away from the circle. The joined fingertips are said to close a particular "circuit" that seals energy in the body. But each finger also has a symbolic meaning: the thumb represents the great self (*parama atman*); the index finger is the embodied self (*jiva atman*); and the three other fingers are the qualities or "strands" (*guna*) — "beingness" (*sattva*), darkness or inertia (*tamas*), and action (*rajas*) — that comprise the material world. So in addition to its practical function, the gesture stamps the practitioner's body with the intention to transcend the limitations of the physical world and unite the great and embodied selves.

Then there are the seals on the other end of the familiarity spectrum, the little-known consciousness (*chitta*) seals. Five of these are included in the *Gheranda-Samhita,* called the Five Concentrations (*pancha dharana*). That leaves the body (*kaya*) seals and their first cousins, the bonds (*bandhas*). Each of my sourcebooks devotes an entire chapter to these practices: Gheranda describes twenty-one seals and four bonds; Svatmarama has six seals and four bonds; and the Anonymous/Shiva teacher discusses eight seals and three bonds. These body seals will be the main focus of this chapter.

Body seals generally involve the eyes, lips, tongue, throat, perineum, and abdomen either individually or in some combination. For all the benefits they're purported to supply to the practitioner, it's a wonder they aren't more widely taught in the West. But in more than thirty years of haunting yoga classes, I can remember only a few times that one of my teachers offered any instruction in these mostly accessible exercises. Of course, it might be that I've been going to the wrong classes all this time or that my teachers, who know the practices perfectly well, are dutifully following the repeated injunctions to keep them strictly secret.

Gheranda notes that the mudras grant us success (*siddhi*) in the world, though as always, his exact meaning isn't clearly defined or, to be kind, is defined very broadly. Svatmarama claims they lead to the eight great powers (see *Origins of Yoga*, preceding chapter 7), and Anonymous/ Shiva credits them with freeing us from disease.

THE SEALS AND BONDS: PRACTICE OVERVIEW

We practiced four mudras as asanas in chapter 5 (Pond, Bird Catcher, two variations of Inverse Action, and Vajroli); Shiva's Seal (*shambhavi mudra*) will be practiced in chapter 8. The remaining twenty exercises (along with a related exercise from the *Hatha-Yoga-Pradipika*) are distributed as follows:

Section 1: The "Winds"
Section 2: Three Bonds (Bandhas)
    Net-Bearing Bond (*jalandhara bandha; Hatha-Yoga-Pradipika*
        3.70–73; *Gheranda-Samhita* 3.10–11; *Shiva-Samhita* 4.60–63)
    Flying-Up Bond (*uddiyana bandha; Hatha-Yoga-Pradipika*
        3.55–60; *Gheranda-Samhita* 3.8–9; *Shiva-Samhita* 4.72–77)
    Root Bond (*mula bandha; Hatha-Yoga-Pradipika* 3.61–69;
        Gheranda-Samhita 3.12–13; *Shiva-Samhita* 4.64–68)
Section 3: Three Greats
    Great Seal (*maha mudra; Hatha-Yoga-Pradipika* 3.10–18;
        Gheranda-Samhita 3.5–6; *Shiva-Samhita* 4.25–36)
    Great Bond (*maha bandha; Hatha-Yoga-Pradipika* 3.19–24;
        Gheranda-Samhita 3.14–16; *Shiva-Samhita* 4.37–42)
    Great Piercer (*maha vedha, Hatha-Yoga-Pradipika* 3.25–29;
        Gheranda-Samhita 3.18–20; *Shiva-Samhita* 4.43–47)

Section 4. Tongue and Lips
  Sky Seal (*nabho mudra; Gheranda-Samhita* 3.7)
  Tongue Bond (*jihva bandha; Hatha-Yoga-Pradipika* 3.22)
  Frog Seal (*manduki mudra; Gheranda-Samhita* 3.51–52)
  Crow Seal (*kaki mudra; Gheranda-Samhita* 3.66)/Serpent Seal
    (*bhujangi mudra Gheranda-Samhita* 3.69–70)
  Little Lamp: Space-Walking Seal (*khechari mudra; Hatha-Yoga-Pradipika* 3.32–55; *Gheranda-Samhita* 3.21–28; *Shiva-Samhita* 5.51–59)
Section 5: Five Concentration Seals (*pancha dharana mudra; Gheranda-Samhita* 3.57–63)
  Earth Concentration Seal (*bhuvodharana mudra; Gheranda-Samhita* 3.59)
  Water Concentration Seal (*varunidharana mudra; Gheranda-Samhita* 3.60)
  Fire Concentration Seal (*vaishvanari dharana mudra, Gheranda-Samhita* 3.61)
  Air Concentration Seal (*vyavi dharana mudra, Gheranda-Samhita* 3.62)
  Ether (or Space) Concentration Seal (*nabhodharana mudra; Gheranda-Samhita* 3.63)
Section 6: Miscellaneous Mudras
  Dawn Horse Seal (*ashvini mudra; Gheranda-Samhita* 3.64)
  Elephant Seal (*matangini mudra; Gheranda-Samhita* 3.67–68)
  Womb Seal (*yoni mudra; Hatha-Yoga-Pradipika* 3.43, *Gheranda-Samhita* 3.33–38; *Shiva-Samhita* 4.2–8)
  Shaking-the-Power Seal (*shakti chalani mudra; Hatha-Yoga-Pradipika* 3.111–119; *Gheranda-Samhita* 3.43-48; *Shiva-Samhita* 4.105–110)

SECTION 1: THE "WINDS" (*VAYU*)

RANA · the breath of life, breath, respiration, spirit, vitality
  (from *pra,* "to fill," and *an,* "to breathe, to live; to move")
VAYU · wind, air; breathing, breath; the wind of the body, a
  vital air (of which five are reckoned, *prana, apana, samana,*

udana, vyana) (from *va*, "to blow," the root of the English
word "wind"); the god of the wind

Before we get to the practice of the seals and bonds, we might ask the
logical question, what are we sealing and bonding? The immediate answer is, of course, the body, and more specifically the torso-pot. But the
answer to the what then leaves us wondering, why? The answer to this
second question takes us right to the heart of Hatha practice, the subtle
"energy" that drives the entire process, usually (but not always) called
prana (see the Little Lamp: *Prana* and its Synonyms).

LITTLE LAMP:
PRANA AND ITS SYNONYMS

My sources use at least nine different words, including *prana* and *vayu*, to
signify our vital energy:

VATA · blown, air (usually refers to the *dosha* responsible for
  movement in the body)

PAVANA · clean, pure, air, wind (from *pu*, "to make clean,
  cleanse, purify," as the wind is said to be able to clean and
  purify

MARUT · wind, air, breeze (from *mri*, "to die," implies that
  when the vital breath is gone, so is life); the name of the
  wind god

ANILA · wind (from *an*, "to breathe")

VAHA · vehicle, that which carries things, as the element of
  air is responsible for moving things around

SAMIRA · air, wind (*samir*, "to shake, move, agitate, stir up,
  set in motion, excite, rouse; send forth, emit")

MAHA KHAGA · literally the "great bird" (from *kha*, "sky;
  heaven"); cavity, hollow; action; knowledge; happiness

I won't say too much here about *prana*, since I've already said pretty
much everything I have to say about it elsewhere. First, there's plenty of
information about *prana* in easily available books and online, and second, in keeping with the down-to-earth approach of this book, I don't

see much purpose in trying to teach much about this presumed subtle energy in a book—I believe that's a job for a living teacher. But from another perspective, it's useful in understanding traditional Hatha Yoga to understand a little about the mechanics of the seals and bonds and how the old yogis used them to work with *prana*.

So cosmic *prana,* once assimilated into the body through inhalation, immediately separates into five major winds (*vayu,* along with five minor winds that won't be part of this discussion), each of which has a special function in our life processes:

PRANA VAYU · forward breath, localized in the chest and responsible for appropriation, that is, taking in (as in inhalation). *Prana vayu*'s natural tendency is to rise (it should not be confused with cosmic *prana;* the former is a modality of the latter).

APANA VAYU · down breath, localized in the pelvis and responsible for elimination, that is, letting go (as in exhalation). *Apana*'s natural tendency is to descend.

SAMANA VAYU · middle breath, localized in the belly (the fire in the belly, *jathara agni*) and responsible for assimilation (as in digestion).

UDANA VAYU · up breath, localized in the throat and responsible for expression.

VYANA VAYU · distributed breath, unlocalized or "distributed" throughout the body and responsible for distribution or circulation of what's been assimilated.

Of these five major *vayus,* only three play an important role in *pranayama*—*prana, apana,* and *samana* (to simplify matters, I'll drop the *-vayu* in the name of each mode from now on)—and of these three, the whole show begins with the first two.

The *vayus* have two functions. To keep us alive is the first and, to a certain extent, the most important, since liberation would be difficult to achieve if we were dead. To serve as transformative agents once the *ghata* is properly prepared is the second function. Cosmic *prana* and *kundalini* are two sides of the same coin: the former is the active world sustaining energy of the goddess; the latter is the dormant key to our ultimate fulfillment, the reason why we're alive at all in that world. To realize that end, we're charged with harnessing and then uniting all our *pranic* forces, using the active side of the goddess to "switch on" her dormant side and so regain, or "unionize," what is for us a divided unity.

This means we first need to bring *prana* and *apana* together. The problem is that the two forces naturally repel each other like the positive ends of a pair of magnets—*prana* tends to rise, while *apana* descends. So the yogis developed Net-Bearing and Root Bonds, not only to seal off the open ends of our *ghata* at the throat and anus, but to move the two energies forcefully in their opposite directions: Net-Bearing forces *prana* downward; Root forces *apana* upward. This pair is then concentrated at the navel and there "heated" with samana, stirred and stoked by compressing the belly through Flying-Up Bond. All of this generates a "fire in the belly" designed to forcefully (*hatha*) awaken the "sleeping" energy, the famous *kundalini.*

Here we have a parable that tells us who we are and where we're headed. We are identified with the slumbering energy, which represents the source of our constant sorrow, our self-forgetfulness of our own authentic self. To wake ourselves up, we're told, we have to conserve all our life energy, prevent it from slipping out and away where it's wasted, and reverse its usual course. We must then concentrate this newly contained energy and heat it with the innate desire we have to know ourselves truly, so that it, in turn, will awaken our authentic self to itself.

SECTION 2. THREE BONDS (BANDHAS)

As noted, the four bonds among the twenty-five exercises in Gheranda's chapter on the seals are, in order of presentation, Flying-Up (*uddiyana*), Net-Bearing (*jalandhara*), Root (*mula*), and Great (*maha*). In Gheranda, the latter two are grouped in a triumvirate with Great Piercer (*maha vedha*), but in Svatmarama, the Great Bond and Great Piercer are grouped with the Great Seal (*maha mudra*). In this practice, we'll follow Svatmarama's lineup and discuss Net-Bearing, Root, and Flying-Up Bonds.

NET-BEARING BOND
(JALANDHARA BANDHA)

JALA · a net (for catching birds, fish, etc.); a snare

DHARA · bearing, supporting, holding, carrying, wearing, possessing, keeping (both in hand and in memory), sustaining, preserving, observing; vein, tubular vessel

Commentators have found several different ways to interpret the Sanskrit word *jalandhara,* which is composed of two shorter words, *jala* and *dhara* (the *n* is inserted when the two are joined for euphonic reasons). Now *jala* (spelled with a long first *a*) means a "net, web, mesh, snare" for catching birds. *Dhara,* as already shown, means "bearing, supporting," as well as "vein" or "tubular vessel" of the body. In this sense, writer Alain Danielou translates *jalandhara* as the "net-holding contraction." He says the bond puts pressure on the purity wheel (*vishuddha chakra*) situated in the throat, which is a kind of command station for the network of "perception-transmitting nerves" in the body, thus protecting the nerve ends "from the brutal pressure of the air while holding the breath."[1]

LITTLE LAMP: *JALA*

Some writers have taken *jala* as spelled with a short first *a,* which changes its meaning to "water" (or any fluid in general). With this spelling, *jalandhara* is defined as the "water-tube bond," which reminds us, as Svatmarama writes (*Hatha-Yoga-Pradipika* 3.71), that the bond also blocks the downward flow of the "water of the sky" (*nabho jala*), the "elixir of immortality." In this context, Theos Bernard defines *jalandhara* as the receptacle of vital fluid,[2] although for some unexplained reason, he also calls it "cloud-holding." In another of his sadly out-of-print books, Bernard mentions that Net-Bearing exercises an upward pull on the spine and spinal cord, which in turn works on the brain. Interpreted in this way, he continues, *jala* refers to the brain and to the nerve (which he doesn't specify) passing through the neck, while *dhara* denotes the upward pull.[3] I haven't been able to discover how he derived these interpretations of the Sanskrit words, though the nerve might be related to what Swami Rama calls the knowledge channel (*vijnani nadi*), or channel of consciousness. According to Rama, Net-Bearing compresses the carotid arteries that feed blood to the brain and brings about a blissful state of mind. Without going into detail, this slows the heartbeat and protects the heart and brain from the great internal pressure of breath retention.[4]

Practice

Jalandhara is often rendered in English as the Throat or Chin Lock, neither of which I favor. "Lock" implies a kind of clamping down that isn't at all desirable in this exercise; I prefer to render *bandha* with the cognate "bond." Further, "chin" emphasizes only half of the performance equation, the other half being the chest or, more specifically, the sternum. In the best of all possible worlds, I'd call this exercise the Chin-Hyoid-Sternum Bond, which emphasizes the importance of focusing on these three bones to create the *bandha*, which helps avoid hardening the throat and/or straining the back of the neck. But this name is a bit too awkward, so we'll just call *jalandhara* by its English translation, Net-Bearing Bond.

Sit in any comfortable sitting pose. The movement of the head is initiated from the base of the skull by lifting the occipital protuberance (the inion) away from the back of the neck. This action draws the crook of the throat (at the hyoid bone) deeper into the head and toward the top of the spine (the atlas). At the same time, the lift of the sternum is initiated by pressing the lower tips of the shoulder blades in and up, that is, diagonally through the upper torso toward the manubrium (top of the sternum). The hyoid serves as a fulcrum for the head, which swivels over it so the chin can lightly meet the manubrium. The crook of the throat is akin to the groins in a standing forward bend: it should feel very "sharp" and deep, so there's no tension in the throat.

It's not advisable to hold Net-Bearing for more than a few breaths at first during *pranayama*. Bring your head up periodically to release any tension in the back of the neck, take a breath or two, then lower your head again.

Traditional Benefit

According to Svatmarama, Net-Bearing "destroys" old age and death. That's because it not only keeps the retained *prana* in the torso, it keeps something very precious *out*—the nectar of immortality (here called *piyusha,* "nectar") that is valued even by the gods. This subtle fluid commonly drips out of its source in the head and is incinerated (and thus wasted) in the "fire" (*vahni*) in the belly. Using Net-Bearing (and probably performing *khechari mudra,* discussed later in this chapter, and traditional Inverse Action Seal), the yogi can preserve and drink *piyusha* to his heart's content.

Both Svatmarama and Gheranda mention that Net-Bearing binds the sixteen *adharas* ("supports, props"), but there's some confusion among my sources on exactly what these are. Several assume that the sixteen are vital points located throughout the body: the toes (or thumbs), ankles, knees, thighs, perineum, genitals, navel, heart, neck, throat, tongue (or palate), nose, midbrow, forehead, head, and fontanel. It might be clear how Net-Bearing affects the points located in and around the throat, but it isn't clear—at least to me—how its influence reaches down to the legs and lower torso. Another source, however, identifies the supports with the sixteen "petals," or energy rays, on the purity wheel (*vishuddha chakra*) located in the throat region. These rays represent "desire, intellect, ego, sound, touch, form, taste, smell, *chitta,* steadfastness, memory, attraction by speech, growth, the subtle body, revivification, and the gross body."[5] Presumably the bond helps the practitioner gain a measure of control over these "energies."

Hint and Caution

If your chin doesn't rest easily on your manubrium, be sure *not* to force them together; instead, slip a rolled-up washcloth under the front of your shirt to support the chin, which will be hold it in place.

ROOT BOND (MULA BANDHA)

> *MULA* · a root (of any plant or tree); figuratively, the foot or lowest part or bottom of anything; basis, foundation, cause, origin, commencement, beginning

The "root" referred to in the name of this bond is the perineum, the fleshy base of the pelvis between the inner thighs and pubic bone in front and the coccyx behind. Gheranda gives slightly different, or maybe more precise, instructions for Root Bond than Svatmarama and the Anonymous/ Shiva do.

Root Bond is best learned from a responsible, experienced teacher. I fear there are way too many inexperienced instructors out there presenting this exercise to their students without understanding its subtleties and dangers. I'll first describe what our traditional teachers have to say, but again, only to give you a taste of the traditional practice. Then I'll give you instructions for what I'd actually like you to do. Why present it this way? Root Bond is typically taught as a forceful contraction of the pelvic floor muscles and the anal sphincter (*ashvini mudra*, see Section 5), which hollows or domes the muscular "root" upward into the pelvis to seal it off. My better-safe-than-sorry approach maintains that Root isn't an exercise that can be learned safely from a book. The modification I'll describe achieves a similar energetic doming of the perineum as a passive response to the actions of surrounding bones. This will give you a feel for Root without creating any muscular disturbances in the pelvic floor.

Traditional Practice: For Your Information Only

Sit in Perfected Pose, one heel pressing against the perineum. Along with the contraction of perineal muscles, Root takes advantage of the pressure of a heel to "plug" the pelvic opening. Forcefully and repeatedly contract the perineum and anus, drawing them upward. Gheranda adds that we should push the "navel knot" (*nabhi granthi*) against the spine (*meru danda*), by which I believe he means to perform Flying-Up Bond.

Modified Practice

To begin, assume a comfortable sitting pose with one heel pressed against the perineum to serve as a tactile aid. The other foot can be inserted between or laid on top of the opposite thigh-calf crease as in Fortunate or Cowherd Pose. Contact the heads of the thighbones and the tailbone, the three points of the sitting tripod, and imagine the bones descending to the floor. Spread the sacrum across the back of the pelvis and narrow the hip points. As the bones drop and narrow, the perineum will ideally "dome" up into the pelvis and feed into the lift of the energetic front spine.

Traditional Benefit

The books agree that Root Bond counters decrepitude (*jara*). Svatmarama adds that it decreases the body's waste products, implying that it improves the assimilation of food and liquid because of intensified gastric fire. But the *Shiva-Samhita* gives the most appealing benefits of this practice: it counters death (*marana*) and contributes to the arousal of *kundalini*. Anonymous/Shiva also states that Root Bond is a preparation for the Womb Seal (*yoni mudra*). By its grace (*prasada*), the yogi conquers the wind (*anila*)—another word for *prana*—and abandons (*utsrijya*) the ground to live in the sky (*gagana*), possibly a reference to the power of levitation or, more realistically, the feeling of physical and psychological lightness that accompanies a successful yoga practice. Finally, echoing Svatmarama in a way, Anonymous/Shiva claims that this bond helps the yogi cross the ocean (*gagara*) or circuit of mundane existence (*samsara*, literally "wandering through") and arrive at self-realization.

Flying-Up Bond (Uddiyana Bandha)

UDDIYANA • flying up, soaring (from *ud*, "upward"; *di*, "to fly"; and *yana*, "conducting, leading")

Like Root Bond, Flying-Up Bond is best learned from an experienced teacher. But it can be practiced with due caution in a sitting pose after some preliminary work while lying supine (face up).

Two things can be thought of as "flying up" in this exercise: one is physical and the other subtle. Outwardly and most noticeably, the abdomen is sucked up and into the torso, radically decreasing its interior volume, through (as we'll do it here) the hydraulic action of the expanded thorax. This in turn squeezes the three *vayus*—prana, apana, and *samana*—that have previously been concentrated at the level of the navel by the Net-Bearing and Root Bonds. Just as a confined gas will heat up if compressed, the combined *vayus*, already "cooking" in the middle breath's digestive fire (which has been purified and intensified by other practices), get hotter and hotter. Eventually the heat will stimulate the dormant spiritual power, making *kundalini* "fly up" through the *sushumna nadi*. For this exercise, you'll need either a block or a thick bolster and a clear wall.

Preliminary Practice

We'll perform this preliminary work in a modified version of *viparita karani mudra*. With your block nearby, sit on the floor with your right side against the wall, knees bent, feet on the floor. Exhale and swing around so your back torso lies on the floor, and lift your legs straight up against the wall. Bend your knees a bit, slide your feet down the wall a foot or so, press your heels against the wall, and lift your pelvis and lower back off the floor. Slide the block under your sacrum at its middle or lowest height, then lower onto the block, and restraighten your legs, sliding your heels up the wall. Your buttocks should be a few inches away from the wall, with your tailbone imaginatively dropping into the space between the block and the wall. Make sure your torso and legs are in alignment, and lay your arms off to the sides, palms up.

For a few minutes, follow your inhalations and exhalations, noting in particular how the rib case expands during the former. In imagining the rib case, I like to picture an umbrella opening (on the inhalation) and closing (on the exhalation), with the imaginary front spine being the umbrella's central shaft and handle. When you have a feel for the movement, exhale fully and take what's been called a "mock inhalation," which means expand your rib case *as if* you're inhaling but don't actually bring in any air. Make sure to expand the back ribs as much as the front—this is where the umbrella image comes in handy for me. Ideally, by opening the rib case without drawing any breath, the front abdomen will hollow between the pubic bone and the lower ribs. Remember: this isn't created by a muscular contraction; it's a passive response to the expanded but uninspired thorax. Hold for maybe 3 to 5 counts at first, then release the ribs and take a few real inhalations. Repeat a few more times. As you gain experience with this exercise over time, you can lengthen the holding time for a few more counts.

Once you've gained some experience in this reclining position, you can try the exercise sitting up. Take your seat for breathing and proceed in the same way as you did when reclining. Watch the breath and ribs first, then perform a mock inhalation. Hold it initially for 3 to 5 counts, and slowly build up your total count to a comfortable number with regular practice over the next few weeks or months.

Traditional Benefit

Svatmarama says that Flying-Up forestalls old age and death if practiced regularly for six months (the *Shiva-Samhita* puts that regularity at four times a day). He calls it the "highest, chief; best, excellent" (*uttama*) of the *bandhas,* and says liberation (*mukti*) will arise naturally or spontaneously (*svabhava*) through its practice.

The *Shiva-Samhita* notes that Flying-Up will do away with "all sorrows" (*sarva duhkha*) and diseases, as well as increase the fire (*agni*) in the belly and the body's essential fluids (*rasa*). All of this will lead to physical perfection (*siddhi*).

Application

These three bonds are used during *pranayama,* which will be described in chapter 7.

SECTION 3: THREE GREATS

What I call the Three Greats are seals with names that all begin with *maha,* meaning "great, mighty": Great Seal (*maha mudra*), Great Bond (*maha bandha*), and Great Piercer (*maha vedha*). In Svatmarama and the *Shiva-Samhita,* they're supposed to be performed in the sequence listed here, whereas Gheranda treats Great Seal separately and begins the sequence with Root Bond (*mula bandha*). We'll follow Svatmarama's sequence. All three, Svatmarama adamantly insists, should be kept in strictest secrecy (*guhya, gopaniya*).

GREAT SEAL (MAHA MUDRA)

MAHA · great, mighty, strong, abundant

Following is an overview of what several different teachers and books say about Great Seal, including Svatmarama, from whom most of the instructions are taken; Gheranda; the *Shiva-Samhita*; the *Hatha-Ratna-Avali*; and the *Hatha-Tatva-Kaumudi*.

Practice

Sit in Staff Pose. Bend your left knee and press your perineum (*yoni*) with the root (*mula*) of your left foot; lay your leg off to the side on the floor. By "root," I believe Svatmarama is referring to the ankle, so you have two choices: you can physically sit on your foot with the ankle (or more likely the inner heel) pressing your perineum, or if that's uncomfortable, sit on the floor or your support and just press your heel against the pubis. Svatmarama calls this position, with the left leg bent, the *chandra* ("moon") side.

Reach out and take the sides of your right foot, either directly with your hands or indirectly with a strap (Gheranda says to grip the *pada angula*, literally the "fingers of the foot," or toes). Keep your arms straight, and by pulling on the foot and firming your shoulder blades against your back, lift the top of your sternum. Take a long, slow inhalation. As you reach the end of the breath, perform Net-Bearing Bond (see Section 2) and—according to Gheranda—Midforehead Gaze (*bhru madhya drishti*). Hold for 5 to 10 counts, then maintaining the Bond, release the breath slowly (never *vega*, or "quickly," according to Svatmarama). At the end of the exhalation, lift your head and take one or more everyday breaths as needed. None of the books say how many times to repeat this breath, but I usually do three repetitions. Be careful here not to overdo the retention time or the number of repetitions. If you get dizzy, please back off and hold the breath for less time and/or reduce the number of repetitions. Now straighten your left leg, square your pelvis, and repeat for the same number of times on the *surya* (sun) side.

The *Shiva-Samhita* adds a couple of interesting instructions. The anonymous teacher tells us to block the "nine doors" (*nava vara*) or openings of the body—the eyes, mouth, ears, nostrils, genitals, and anus. The first two are "blocked" by closing the eyelids and lips respectively, the last two by the ankle or heel, and the rest by imaginatively drawing the normally outgoing senses of hearing and smelling inward, just as the Tortoise pulls its limbs into its shell. You might recognize this as sense withdrawal (*pratyahara*), the fifth limb of Patanjali's Ashtanga Yoga. Anonymous/Shiva tells us, somewhat cryptically, to then direct our consciousness (*chitta*) along the "path of consciousness" (*chitta patha*). What does this mean? My understanding is that once the senses are interiorized, consciousness follows. I believe the path of consciousness is the route consciousness followed as it evolved from the Source into the world. Through intense meditation, it would be possible to retrace this route back to the Source.

Traditional Benefit

The benefits afforded by Great Seal, if we accept them at face value, are truly amazing. Indeed, the *Shiva-Samhita* feels it's necessary to assure us that they're not to be doubted (*vichara*). No wonder the yogis wanted to keep it a secret. Or from a different perspective, we might ask why, when they had this life-transforming, world-saving technique at their disposal, they weren't willing to share it with society at large. Maybe they shared their wisdom sub rosa, because they were concerned that if the cat were let out of the bag completely, the techniques would be exploited by unscrupulous individuals preying on the naive.

In general, according to several sources, this exercise can cure great yet unnamed afflictions (*maha klesha*), unnamed deficiencies (*dosha*), and diseases such as leprosy (*kushtha*) and enlarged spleen. It will let you drink the most venomous poison (*visha, kalakuta*) as if it were nectar (*piyusha*) — kids, *don't* try this at home. It will stoke your digestive fires (*jathara agni*) and give you tremendous strength (*bala*) and personal power (*siddhi*). It will expiate sins (*pataca*), which I prefer to interpret as restoration of "loss of caste"; help you achieve all your goals; and provide you with "comfort, happiness, enjoyment" (*saukhya*). Enough? Not done yet. It can reverse the aging process, darkening gray hair (*palita*) in the process, and even eliminate (or perhaps better, forestall) death (*marana, mrita*). Finally, through Great Seal, you can purify your subtle energy channels (*nadis*); direct *prana* to the "Brahma hole" (*brahma randhra;* see chapter 8); and icing on the cake, stimulate slumbering *kundalini.*

GREAT BOND (MAHA BANDHA)

Our revered teachers were mostly on the same page when it came to the practice of Great Seal. But now we have two camps regarding Great Bond, so once again, we'll take our lead from Svatmarama.

Practice

As you did with Great Seal, press the left ankle or heel against the perineum (*yoni sthana,* literally "source place"), then bring the right leg into Half-Lotus. This position can also be thought of as a modified Hero Pose (Gheranda says to sit in Perfected Pose). Inhale fully, perform Net-Bearing Bond and Root Bond as in Section 2, and fix the mind (*manas*) in the middle (*madhya*)—that is, the *sushumna nadi.* (As an aside, the *Hatha-Ratna-Avali* says to inhale through the mouth, the only book to do so). Svatmarama says to hold the breath as long as possible, but 5 to 10 counts should be sufficient.

What happens next is described here only to give you a sense of the source practice. I'm not suggesting you try to disturb any "sleeping serpents" based on instructions in this or any other book. For that, you'll need an experienced teacher to supervise and monitor your actions.

That said, according to the *Shiva-Samhita,* while retaining the breath, contract both the anus and the perineum—meaning, perform Root Bond and move the *apana vayu* upward. Simultaneously, apply Net-Bearing Bond to move the *prana vayu* downward (*adho mukha,* "face down"). Join the rising *apana* and descending *prana* with the *samana* ("middle breath"; see Section 1). These concentrated energies generate tremendous physical and psychic heat, the aim being to awaken the slumbering serpent in the root chakra and lead her upward through the *sushumna nadi* to the head (*murdha*), or more particularly, the crown center.

Getting back to the real instructions, exhale slowly (*shana*). Once again, there's no indication of how many times to repeat the exercise, so I usually do two or three repetitions. Go back to neutral, reverse the position of the legs, and do the same number of repetitions on the opposite side. As he did with the six acts, Svatmarama notes a disagreement among the teachers, this time regarding Net-Bearing Bond. It's better, according to the dissenters, to press the tongue against the front teeth (*raja danta*, literally the "king teeth") and avoid Net-Bearing.

Traditional Benefit

The benefits attributed to Great Bond are no less amazing than those assigned to Great Seal. It beautifies (*vapusha*) and nourishes (*pushti*) the body; firmly binds the skeleton (*panjara*); confers great power so the yogi can achieve whatever he wants in the "three worlds" (*tri bhuvana*, meaning earth, sky, and heaven); halts the aging process (*jara*) and loosens the "noose" (*bandha*) of the rope of time (*kala pasha*); directs *prana* (or "wind," *vayu*) into *sushumna nadi*. It ultimately causes the consciousness to reach *kedara* (literally a "field" or "meadow," a symbolic pilgrimage site in the human body) identified with the *shiva sthana* ("Shiva's Place"; see Chapter 7), the holiest place in our body (also called the *tri vena*, the "triple knot," where the three main *nadis* come together at the "third eye"), or Shiva's Himalayan mountain home.

GREAT PIERCER (MAHA VEDHA)

VEDHA · penetrating, piercing, breaking through; breach, opening, perforation (from *vyadh*, "to pierce")

To encourage the performance of the third member of the Great trio, both Gheranda and Svatmarama make a comment that wouldn't sit well with most female students nowadays. Of course, we have to account for the different times and cultures and cut our ancients a bit of slack. Without this seal, say our two revered teachers, Great Seal and Great Bond are like a beautiful woman without a man. Ouch!

Once all that energy is stirred up and concentrated at the navel by the first two exercises, what's needed is a little tap on the bottom to get it moving upward.

Practice: Svatmarama's Practice

Sit in Great Bond, inhale, apply Net-Bearing Bond, and fix your consciousness on one thought (*dhi*, "especially a religious thought, meditation, devotion; wisdom"). Press both hands on the floor beside your hips, and slowly bounce your buttocks on the floor. Svatmarama says the breath now enters the middle (*madhya*), which is always a code word for *sushumna nadi*. None of our teachers specifies exactly how many times to do this, so I usually bounce somewhere between five and eight times, first with the legs one way, then for the same number of times with the legs reversed. The *Shiva-Samhita* remarks that these three exercises are to be practiced four times a day, presumably every six hours, at dawn, noon, twilight, and midnight. For our purposes, once a day (or at least regularly) will be sufficient.

Traditional Benefit

The *Shiva-Samhita* asserts that the practitioner will overcome death after six months (of presumably regular) practice. Svatmarama seconds this (though he doesn't mention a time frame) and adds that Great Piercer confers great powers, reverses the aging process, and stokes the digestive fire (*vahni*).

Application

I use the Three Greats as a preparation for *pranayama*.

SECTION 4: TONGUE AND LIPS

This section covers four traditional exercises, three for the tongue and one for the lips.

SKY SEAL (NABHO MUDRA)

> **NABHA** · sky, atmosphere (denotes "bursting forth" or "expanding")

Curl the tongue up and back toward the soft palate at the back of the mouth. This exercise is a precursor to *khecahari mudra*. I use it in conjunction with the Lion's "roar." Try this. As you inhale, curl your tongue back and touch its tip as close as you can to the soft palate. Then with a Lion exhalation, stretch the tongue out. Repeat several times — inhaling/curling, exhaling/stretching.

Traditional Benefit

This practice destroys all disease.

TONGUE BOND (JIHVA BANDHA)

> JIHVA · the tongue or tongues of Agni, that is, various forms
> of flame; also identified with the seven winds (*prana, apana,*
> *udana, samana, vyana, paryana, nivahana*); the tongue of a
> balance; speech

Practice

Press the upper surface of the tongue firmly against the root of the front teeth.

Traditional Benefit

Used as an alternative to Net-Bearing Bond, this bond stops the upward course of the *prana* through all the *nadis* except *sushumna* and exercises the neck muscles.

LITTLE LAMP: TONGUE BOND

While researching *jihva bandha,* I ran across an interesting idea. We all have an inner voice that talks to us almost continually during the day. Apparently while we're "talking to ourselves," we activate the same muscle — the tongue — that we use when talking to others. The tongue movement in self-talk isn't as obvious as it is in "other-talk," but the tongue still makes micromovements that activate speech-supporting muscles in the lips and face.

You can turn all this around to quiet your internal talk. First soften your jaw, then perform what's essentially *jihva bandha.* This prevents your tongue from making its micromovements, softens the muscles of your face, and (to some degree) placates the chatterbox in your head. (See, for example, "Eliminating Anxiety and Panic Attacks" by Vincent Harris at http://panic-attacks-treatment-advice.com/blog/eliminating-anxiety-and-panic-attacks-by-vincent-harris.)

FROG SEAL (MANDUKI MUDRA)

Practice

Close the mouth and slowly move the root of the tongue around. Though he doesn't say so directly, I believe Gheranda means to circularly massage the soft palate at the back of the mouth (at least this interpretation of the exercise is most useful for me). I like to circle slowly in one direction for 30 seconds to a minute, then reverse the circle for about the same length of time. Gheranda then says to drink the elixir of immortality, the flow of which is presumably stimulated by the pressure of the tongue.

Traditional Benefit

This practice removes wrinkles (*vali*) and gray hair and bestows "eternal youth" (*nitya yauvana*).

CROW SEAL (KAKI MUDRA) / SERPENT SEAL (BHUJANGI MUDRA)

> **KAKA** · crow (perhaps an onomatopoeic imitation of the cawing of the crow)
>
> **BHUJAGA** · "going in curves"; serpent, snake

These two practices seem closely related: both involve pursing the lips as if in an exaggerated kiss. We'll focus here on *kaki mudra*.

Practice

For *kaki mudra*, shape the mouth like a crow's beak and slowly suck in air. This can be used as alternative to the rolled-up tongue in Cooling breath (*shitali pranayama*, see chapter 7).

Traditional Benefit

Kaki destroys all disease, while *bhujangi* cures tummy ailments, especially indigestion.

LITTLE LAMP: THE SPACE-WALKING SEAL
(KHECHARI MUDRA)

KHA · cavity, hollow, cave, cavern, aperture; an aperture of
the human body (of which there are nine: the mouth, the
ears, the eyes, the nostrils, the anus, and the genitals); the
hole in the nave of a wheel through which the axis runs;
vacuity, empty space, air, ether, sky

CARA · moving, walking, wandering

Among the several strange practices developed by the yogis over the centuries, *khechari mudra* is no doubt among the top three. One of the main goals of Hatha Yoga is to extend life well beyond the normal span of years, and to do that, as we've seen, the yogis try to preserve their internal supply of *amrita*. But they also try to increase the supply, to ensure that they have a reserve to draw on when needed. Although the old books aren't consistent on this, the source of the fluid seems to be somewhere in the head. The yogis directly stimulate this center with their tongue, though if you've ever tried to reach back under your soft palate with your tongue, you know that it's normally way too short. So (if you're squeamish, you may want to skip the rest of this paragraph) to stretch his tongue, the yogi first cuts the frenum, the flap of skin that anchors it to the floor of his mouth. Next he uses a special pair of tongs to pull and stretch the muscle regularly until he can touch the tip to the bridge of his nose. With this Gene Simmons–like tongue, the yogi can now stimulate his *amrita* source whenever he likes.

SECTION 5: FIVE CONCENTRATION SEALS
(PANCHA DHARANA MUDRA)

DHARANA · holding, keeping (in remembrance), retaining, preserving, protecting; assuming the shape of, resembling; immovable concentration of the mind on; collection
or concentration of the mind (joined with the retention of
breath); firmness, righteousness

The five concentrations upon the elements [respectively have the power of] stopping, inundating, burning, destabilizing, and dessicating. . . . The Yogin who is intelligent [in the use of these techniques] is released from all suffering.

— *Goraksha-Paddhati 2.59–60 (translation by Georg Feuerstein)*

Earlier in this chapter, I made mention of the category of mudras known as consciousness seals (*chitta mudras*), a sequence of five of which is described by Gheranda. Unlike the physical seals of the hands and body, consciousness seals are visualizations that focus on specific areas in the body. In the *Gheranda-Samhita,* the visualized seals are located in the heart, throat, palate, midbrow, and crown, though in other books the locales may be different (for example, see *Shiva-Samhita* 3.72–78).

The first four visualization seals are distinguished by a particular geometric shape and color (the last, ether, is unique), each of them representing a corresponding traditional element; for example, a yellow square represents the earth element. Remember that these yoga elements aren't found on the periodic table alongside oxygen and molybdenum. They're thought of, instead, as "crystalizations" of various frequencies of subtle vital energy (*prana*). Along with shapes and colors, each center also has a particular "seed" syllable (*bija*) or mantra, as well as a presiding male deity (*deva*).

The concentration seals are arranged here by their corresponding elements in order of density, beginning with the densest (earth) and ending with the most subtle (ether or space). The pictorial representation of each presiding deity is complicated and highly symbolic, so all I'll give you here is his name (along with, just to be fair, his traditional female counterpart). If you want a fuller account of the deities' appearances and symbolism to enhance your visualization, consult any of the following:

Alain Danilou, *The Gods of India* (Inner Traditions, 1985)
Swami Sivananda Radha, *Kundalini Yoga for the West*
   (Shambhala, 1981)
Arthur Avalon, *The Serpent Power* (Dover, 1974)

Traditional Benefit

By mastering these concentrations, nothing in existence is impossible (except perhaps for the Cubs to win the World Series). The yogi can travel through space (*kha*) as fast as thought and go to heaven (*svarga*) while still in his human body.

Practice

The sequence begins with concentration on the yoga heart and slowly works upward through the throat, palate, and forehead, ending at the crown. We're asked to center our breath at each station in turn and, at the same time, visualize the corresponding colored shape and deity (we'll forgo the latter) and repeat its seed (*bija*) syllable. In this way, we can potentially create and experience different states or qualities of consciousness; for example, if an apocalyptic hurricane huffs and puffs at your door — maybe in the form of some unsettling news — and threatens to blow your house down, you might work with the earth center to establish stability in the face of uncertainty.

The specific instructions are the same for each concentration. Gheranda tells us to hold the visualization and breath in each center for 5 *ghatikas* (1 *ghatika* equals 24 minutes), or 2 hours. I assume that, like me, you don't have a spare 10 hours during the average day to dedicate to this sequence. I'm pretty sure, though, that you can find the time to visit each center for 3 to 5 minutes, sufficient time — I hope — to help you through your next personal *pralaya*. To begin, sit in a comfortable yoga asana, close your eyes, and direct your awareness inward

EARTH CONCENTRATION SEAL

BHUMI · earth, soil, ground

The earth element is situated at the yoga heart, which is in the center of the chest (the physical heart, of course, is slightly to the left). It's represented by a "brilliant" (*rucira*) yellow square that signifies strength, firmness, solidity, and cohesion; its seed syllable is LA; and its presiding deities are Brahma and Dakini (or Savitri).

Traditional Benefit

Earth concentration leads to "strength" (*stambha*).

LITTLE LAMP: LA, VA, RA, YA

The first four seed mantras in this practice are what Sanskrit calls the semivowels. Like the entire Sanskrit alphabet (or syllabary), these phonemes comprise a sophisticated philosophical system far beyond the scope of this book, not to mention its author. Suffice it to say that all four tell a story of the encounter between the power of will (*iccha*) or awakening (*unmesa*) and the Absolute, resulting in various qualities like immobility (earth) and heat (fire). For all the information you'll ever want to know about this subject, see the chapter titled "The Phonematic Emanation" in *Vac: The Concept of the Word in Selected Hindu Tantras* by André Padoux.

WATER CONCENTRATION SEAL

AMBHAS · water, the celestial waters; power, fruitfulness; collective name for gods, humans, and *asuras*

The water element is situated at the throat (*kantha*). It's represented by a half moon, white as a jasmine flower. Its seed syllable is VA (a name of Varuna, which means "ocean, water"), and its presiding deities are Vishnu and Rakini.

Traditional Benefit

Water concentration alleviates suffering (*tapas*, "consumed by heat") and sin (*papa*). It's noted elsewhere that if you master this seal, you'll never be able to drown, even in the deepest water. Sundara Deva notes that through mastery of this element, the practitioner will gain power over speech (*Hatha-Tatva-Kaumudi* 47.10).

FIRE CONCENTRATION SEAL

VAISHVANARA · relating or belonging to all men, omnipresent, known or worshipped everywhere, universal, general, common, complete; relating or belonging to the gods collectively; all-commanding; relating or sacred to Agni; the fire of digestion; the sun, sunlight; name of the Supreme Spirit or Intellect when located in a supposed collective aggregate of gross bodies (from *vishva,* "all, whole, entire, universal," and *nara,* "a person")

The Fire element is situated at the palate. It's represented by an inverted triangle, blazing red like the cochineal or Indragopa insect (literally "protected by Indra"), whose crushed and dried body is used to make red dye. Its seed syllable is RA ("fire, heat"), and its presiding deities are Rudra ("crying, howling, roaring, dreadful, horrible") and Lakini.

Traditional Benefit

Fire Concentration Seal alleviates, in Gheranda's words, *kala gabhira bhiti harani,* or the "deep, black dread of death." It's noted elsewhere that if you master this seal, you can be tossed into a roaring fire and you won't burn up. Sundara Deva notes that through mastery of this element, the practitioner will be able to enter another body (*Hatha-Tatva-Kaumudi* 47.10).

AIR CONCENTRATION SEAL

VAYAVA · relating or belonging to the wind or air; given by
or sacred to the god of wind

The air element is situated between the eyebrows. It's represented by a circle that resembles a mass of lampblack. Its seed syllable is YA, and its presiding deities are Ishvara (or Isha, "lord") and Kakini.

LITTLE LAMP: *ANJANA*

The word used for "lampblack" here is *anjana,* which has a number of suggestive interpretations: "act of applying an ointment or pigment, embellishing, black pigment or collyrium applied to the eyelashes or the inner coat of the eyelids; a special kind of this pigment, as lampblack, antimony; paint, especially as a cosmetic; magic ointment; ink; night."

Traditional Benefit

Air Concentration Seal allows you to move through space (*kha*). It's noted elsewhere that if you master this seal, you needn't fear death from aerial accidents.

ETHER (OR SPACE) CONCENTRATION SEAL (NABHODHARANA MUDRA)

AKASHA • free or open space, vacuity; ether, sky, or atmosphere; the subtle and ethereal fluid (supposed to fill and pervade the universe and to be the peculiar vehicle of life and sound); Brahma (as identical to ether)

The space element is situated at the crown (the *brahma randhra,* "Brahma opening") and looks like "pure rain" (*vishuddha varisa*). Its seed syllable is HA (*ha,* a name of a form of Shiva, as well as "cipher; meditation, auspiciousness, sky, heaven; blood, dying, fear; knowledge; moon; war; pride; cause, motive"), and its presiding deities are Sada-shiva (or Ardha Narishvara, who's androgynous, with a male right half and a female left half—the female goddess Uma, who's also called Parvati and Durga) and Shakini.

Traditional Benefit

Space Concentration is said to break down the "doorway to liberation." It's also noted that the yogi who practices this seal is untouched by "old age and death."

SECTION 6: MISCELLANEOUS MUDRAS

The descriptions of these mudras are for reading interest only. I *don't* recommend practicing them without expert supervision.

Dawn Horse Seal (Ashvini Mudra)

ASHVIN · possessed of or consisting of horses; mounted on horseback; a cavalier; horse tamer; the two charioteers, two divinities who appear in the sky before the dawn in a golden carriage drawn by horses or birds (they bring treasures to men and avert misfortune and sickness; they are considered the physicians of heaven)

According to Georg Feuerstein, this seal is named after the Ashvins, the golden twin charioteers who, according to Vedic mythology, pulled their sister Usha's chariot at dawn.

Practice

Contract and dilate the anal sphincter muscle repeatedly.

Traditional Benefit

This seal invigorates the body; cures diseases of the rectum; and helps awaken *kundalini,* or *shakti.*

Elephant Seal (Matangini Mudra)

Practice

Stand in neck-deep water. First draw in water through the nostrils and expel it out the mouth; then draw in water through the mouth and expel it through the nostrils.

Traditional Benefit

This seal destroys decay and death; it also confers great strength "like an elephant."

Womb Seal (Yoni Mudra)

YONI · womb, uterus, female organs of generation; a typical symbol of the divine procreative energy; place of birth, source, fountain (sprung or produced from); place of rest, seat, abode

Nowadays a modified version of *yoni mudra* is known as the "six-openings seal" (*shan mukhi mudra;* see *Light on Yoga* #46). In the *Hatha-Yoga-Pradipika, yoni mudra* is another term for *vajroli mudra.*

Practice: Gheranda's Version

Sit in Perfected Pose. Block the ear holes with the thumbs (pressing on the tragi, as described in chapter 2) and the eyes with the index fingers; block the nostrils halfway with the middle fingers and the mouth with the ring and little fingers. Inhale with Crow Seal (see Section 4), meditate on the six chakras in succession using the mantras HUM and HAMSA (see chapter 7) and imagine raising the "sleeping serpent" from her residence in the base of the spine to join with Shiva at the crown. Then say to yourself, "I am Brahman."

LITTLE LAMP: HUM

The mantra HUM is called the "armor seed [mantra]" (*kavacha bija*). It means, "May I be protected" (for more detail about HAMSA, see chapter 7).

Practice: Anonymous/Shiva's Version

Fix your attention in the root chakra at the base of the pelvis, and perform Root Bond. Meditate on the god of love (*kama*), who happens to be shaped like a ball (*kanduka;* some translations interpret this as *bandhuka,* a flower) that looks like ten million (*koti*) suns and ten million moons. Above this, visualize the "highest digit" (*parama kala*), or a "subtle flame" (*shikha,* or "ray of light"), whose form is consciousness (*cidrupa*). Imagine joining with this flame. The visualization continues from here, but this should be enough for the time being.

Traditional Benefit

Practitioners of this seal are never polluted by sins.

SHAKING-THE-POWER SEAL (SHAKTI CHALANI MUDRA)

> *SHAKTI* · power, ability, strength, might, effort, energy,
> capability, faculty, skill, capacity for; effectiveness or
> efficacy (of a remedy); regal power (consisting of three
> parts: *prabhutva,* "personal preeminence," *mantra,* "good
> counsel," and *utsaha,* "energy"); the energy or active power
> of a deity personified as his wife and worshipped by the
> Shaktas, a sect of Hindus, under various names; the power,
> force, or most effective word of a sacred text or magic for-
> mula; the creative power or imagination (of a poet); help,
> aid, assistance, gift, bestowal
>
> *CALA* · moving, trembling, shaking

Practice: Gheranda's Version

Sit in Perfected Pose. Rub the body with ashes and wrap the waist with
a soft, white cloth, 9 inches long and 3 inches wide, held in place with a
tied string. Restrain and join the *prana* and *apana vayus,* perform *ashvini
mudra,* and force (*hatha*) the air to enter *sushumna.*

Practice: Anonymous/Shiva's Version

Anonymous/Shiva is a bit vague on the nuts and bolts of this practice.
He tells us to sit in Freedom Pose and continue the work for 2 *muhur-
tas,* 96 minutes. We're supposed to "agitate, shake" (*cala*) the *kundalini*
sleeping in the "base lotus" (*adhara kamala*) and force (*bala*) her up
sushumna nadi. Here you see a good example of why the overall practice
is called *Hatha* Yoga.

Traditional Benefit

Stirring–the-Power Seal is said to be a preparation for Womb Seal. It
supposedly causes the *kundalini* to "breathe hard" (*shvasa*) and forces
it to enter the "upward path" (*urdhva marga*), meaning *sushumna nadi.*

Turn Out the Light

Certain schools of practice define the mudra symbolically, reminding us that all the exercises of every kind always have, besides their physical expression, a spiritual dimension. So in this case, a mudra is that which brings us joy (*muda*), melts our bondage (*mu*), or seals up the entire universe in the condition of liberation. Jaideva Singh quotes the great Kashmiri philosopher Abhinava Gupta: "That which enables living beings to acquire Self-Realization in all the states [i.e., waking, dream, dreamless deep sleep] of the embodied one is a Mudra."[6]

7

—— ❦ ——

PRANAYAMA

PRA · forth, away

AN · to breathe, to respire; to live; to move,
to go (from the Latin *animus*, "soul, spirit," and
English "animal, equanimity, unanimous")

AYAMA · stretching, extending; restraining,
restrained, stopping

PRANAYAMA IS LITERALLY the "extension and restraint of the 'breathing forth,'"—that is, the breath, which is the most accessible manifestation of the subtle *prana*. *Prana* has this dual reference, to the gross breath and to subtle vital energy. I've written extensively on *pranayama* in two other books, so I'll keep this chapter fairly short and basic, though that doesn't mean I'm minimizing the importance of *pranayama* in traditional Hatha Yoga.

Why do we want to practice *pranayama*? Svatmarama opens his chapter on the subject by citing two major reasons. First, he says, breath and consciousness (*chitta*) are intimately related; we'd say they're two sides of the same coin. Our efforts to realize the traditional goal of our practice—the reorientation of our identity with our authentic self—are for naught if consciousness is unstable, or as Svatmarama says, "trembling" (*chala*, "shaking, fluctuating, disturbed, unsteady, confused, agitated"). It's possible but difficult to work with consciousness directly; it's much easier to approach it indirectly through the breath, which is far more tangible. So steady (*nishchala*) the breath, says the ever-pragmatic Svatmarama, and we can steady consciousness, which results in a steady (*sthana*) yogi.

Moreover, if we're ever to gain this kind of self-identification, we need to practice regularly, and to do that—I suppose I'm stating the obvious—we need to be alive. The yogis have an unusual way of measuring life, not by years, but by number of breaths. They believe that each of us has a certain stockpile of breaths allotted to us, and when we use them up, our time on earth is up. If you accept this premise, it stands to reason that the faster we breathe, the faster we use up our breath allotment and the sooner we die; but the slower we breathe, the longer we'll live. Long life is highly desirable for most of us, though I don't think we could articulate why. The yogis want to prolong their lives for two specific reasons: first, a long life gives them more time to practice, and more practice gets them ever closer to their goal of liberation; and second, if they do happen to reach their goal, long life let's them enjoy their liberated existence. This is called *jivan mukti*, "embodied freedom," the condition of the universe-roaming perfected ones (*maha siddhas*) that Svatmarama catalogs at *Hatha-Yoga-Pradipika* 1.5–9.

Why practice *pranayama*? Apparently, after all the work we've done with the six acts and the asanas, the *nadis* are still clogged with dirt (*mala*) and need further flushing out. This is accomplished with a breathing practice Gheranda calls *nadi shuddhi* ("cleansing, purification, holiness; setting free, rendering secure; justification, quittance, clearing off or paying off; verification, genuineness, truth; clearness, certainty"). Notice that, as usual, the physical practice has psychological and spiritual implications: the purification of the subtle energy channels implies not only innocence, clarity, and truth, but holiness as well.

PRANAYAMA PRACTICE OVERVIEW

Our two yogis each describe eight *pranayamas*, though both call them *kumbhakas*, "potlike," the word we typically use nowadays for breath retention. This emphasizes the central importance of this practice in the Hatha tradition (and the corresponding importance of the Three

Bonds crucial for the retention and transformation of the breath/*prana:* Net-Bearing, Root, and Flying-Up). We'll start in Section 1 with *nadi shuddhi,* which neither of our yogis consider a formal *pranayama;* though the first *pranayama* on Gheranda's list is Accompanied Pranayama (*sahita pranayama*), which is similar to and consequently will be paired with *nadi shuddhi.* Of the eight *pranayamas* in each book, six are common to both yogis (see *Hatha-Yoga-Pradipika* 2.44 and *Gheranda-Samhita* 5.46), and four of these serve as the topic of Section 2. Gheranda's Absolute (*kevala*) Pranayama is the subject of Section 3, and the remaining four practices are briefly described, though not practiced, in Section 4.

Section 1: Purification
    Purification of the Channels (*nadi shuddhi; Hatha-Yoga-Pradipika* 2.7–10; *Gheranda-Samhita* 5.37–45)
    Accompanied Pranayama (*sahita pranayama; Gheranda-Samhita* 5.47–54)
Section 2: Four Pranayamas
    Conqueror (*ujjayi; Hatha-Yoga-Pradipika* 2.51–53; *Gheranda-Samhita* 5.64–67)
    Unwhispered Mantra (*ajapa mantra*)
    Ratio Breathing
    Sun Piercing (*surya bhedana; Hatha-Yoga-Pradipika* 2.48–50; *Gheranda-Samhita* 5.58–63)
    Bee (*bhramari; Hatha-Yoga-Pradipika* 2.68; *Gheranda-Samhita* 5.73–77)
    Cooling (*shitali; Hatha-Yoga-Pradipika* 2.56-58; *Gheranda-Samhita* 5.68–69)
Section 3: Retention (*kumbhaka*)
    Little Lamp: Unaccompanied Retention (*kevala kumbhaka; Hatha-Yoga-Pradipika* 2.71–74; *Gheranda-Samhita* 5.79–91)
Section 4: Miscellaneous Pranayamas
    Bellows (*bhastrika; Hatha-Yoga-Pradipika* 2.60–67; *Gheranda-Samhita* 5.71–72)
    Swooning (*murchchha; Hatha-Yoga-Pradipika* 2.69; *Gheranda-Samhita* 5.78)

Sit [Sound] Making (*sitkari; Hatha-Yoga-Pradipika* 2.54–55)
Floating (*plavini; Hatha-Yoga-Pradipika* 2.70)

Traditional Benefit

Svatmarama says that *pranayama,* if practiced appropriately (*yukta*), will weaken (*kshaya*) disease. But if it is practiced inappropriately, it will strengthen disease, possibly causing hiccups (*hikka*); asthma (*shvasa*); and head (*shira*), ear (*karna*), and eye (*aksha*) pain (*vedana*). With proper practice, the body will be "lean" (*krishata*) and "bright" like the moon (*kanta*). Gheranda claims that by mastering this practice, we become *deva tulya,* "comparable to a god" (*Gheranda-Samhita* 5.1). He adds to Svatmarama's benefits that the yogi gains the ability to move through space (*kha*), becomes happy (*sukha*), and awakens *shakti*.

SECTION 1: PURIFICATION

PURIFICATION OF THE CHANNELS (NADI SHUDDHI)

You might be familiar with the traditional *pranayama* practice called alternate-nostril breathing. Originally it was known as *nadi shuddhi,* but in the *Gheranda-Samhita,* it's considered a preparation for the practice, a means of "purifying" the *nadis* but not a formal *pranayama.* However, there is a practice called *sahita pranayama* that outwardly mimics *nadi shuddhi,* the difference between the two being the accompanying visualizations and mantras. Here I'll briefly describe both and leave it up to you whether, in a modified form, you want to use the practice as a preparation or formal *pranayama.*

There are two types of *nadi shuddhi:* "with thinking" (*samanu*), that is, breathing with a seed syllable or mantra; and "without thinking" (*nirmanu*), which isn't *pranayama* at all but simply the six acts we covered in chapter 3. It seems that either of these practices were considered effective as warm-ups for *pranayama. Nirmanu* won't concern us here.

Nadi shuddhi belongs to the category of digital breathing, which means the breath through the nose is regulated by pressing on the nostrils with the fingertips. One hand, usually the right, is shaped into what's called the Doe Seal (*mrigi mudra*), and the fingertips are used to alternately close one nostril while the breath is being inhaled or exhaled through the other open one. While modern schools may differ on the pattern (which nostril should be open first?), traditionally the inhalation/exhalation pattern is as follows:

> Right nostril blocked — inhale left
> Left nostril blocked — exhale right
> Left nostril blocked — inhale right
> Right nostril blocked — exhale left

Technically, each breathing cycle consists of four phases, though Gheranda only recognizes three: inhalation, internal retention (*antara kumbhaka*), and exhalation. (There should be a fourth phase called external retention, or *bahya kumbhaka*). The phases of each breathing cycle are adjusted according to a set ratio, 1 count inhalation, 4 counts internal retention, 2 counts exhalation (that is, 1:4:2); we should add 1 count external retention (making the four-phase ratio 1:4:2:1). In other words, if we take a 16-count inhalation (which we won't) as Gheranda instructs, the internal retention would last 64 counts, the exhalation 32, and the external retention 16.

It's not clear from the instructions if each phase has a seed mantra and visualization or not, and because it seems so haphazard and confusing, I won't include those instructions here.

LITTLE LAMP: HOW LONG?

We're told we can purify our energy channels with *nadi shuddhi*, but it's not clear exactly how long that will take. I did a little calculating based on the instructions laid out by Svatmarama:

Number of practices a day	4 (sunrise, noon, sunset, midnight)
Number of rounds each practice	80
Total number of rounds each day	320
Length of each round	112 counts (inhale for 16 counts, retain for 64 counts, exhale for 32 counts)

Length of each count	Approximately 1 second (probably a bit longer)
Total time each practice round	About 2.5 hours (4 rounds per day)
Total practice time each day	About 10 hours
Recommended length of regular practice	3 months (about 90 days)
Total practice time	900 hours

ACCOMPANIED PRANAYAMA (SAHITA PRANAYAMA)

> SAHITA · joined, conjoined, united; accompanied
> or attended by, associated or connected with,
> possessed of

After spending nine verses on *nadi shuddhi*, Gheranda turns immediately to *sahita pranayama*, the first of eight traditional breaths. I should note that just as Gheranda doesn't call his practice Hatha Yoga, neither does he call the breathing exercises *pranayama*; rather, he labels them *kumbhaka* (potlike), another reference to the *ghata* torso where the *pranic* energy is restrained and transformed. The word emphasizes the central importance of retention to this practice.

Except for differences in visualizations and mantras, *sahita* is patterned exactly like *nadi shuddhi*. The inhalation, retention, and exhalation are again "accompanied" with visualizations—of deities (Brahma, Vishnu, and Shiva); qualities (*guna*); and colors (red, black, white)—and *bija* mantras (the three constituents of OM, *a-u-m*).

LITTLE LAMP: OM

Perhaps the most famous of all Hindu mantras is OM, often called the *mula mantra*, the "root mantra," because it's believed that all other mantras emerge from it. We're accustomed to seeing it spelled "*o-m*," but in fact, it is composed of three letters: *a, u,* and *m*. These three have myriad associations with deities, the Sanskrit alphabet, time and space, books of the Veda—you name it. But because of the "junction" (*sandhi*) rules of Sanskrit grammar, when a *u* follows an *a,* the two letters blend and become an *o.*

Gheranda instructs us to sit in Lotus Pose (*padmasana*) on a seat (*asana*) covered with kusha grass (optional) and an antelope or tiger skin — which we'll replace with a blanket in deference to antelopes and tigers — facing either east or north. For the time being, we'll forgo the visualizations and mantras, and just focus on the breath.

Hand Mudra

The hand mudra used to manipulate the nostrils is traditionally made with the right (*dakshina,* also "able, clever, dextrous") hand, though I have no objections to southpaws using their dominant hand (*vama,* "left," but also "adverse, contrary, unfavorable; wicked, base, low, bad). Typically the gesture involves the thumb, ring, and little fingers; the index and middle fingers are burrowed into the mound of the thumb. Beginners often have a difficult time forming this hand position because the ring finger is supposed to lap over its diminutive neighbor, the two fingertips lining up to make a single surface. But try as it might, the ring finger just can't seem to curl easily into place at first. If you find this to be a problem, don't worry; just use the thumb and ring finger for your practice until you can manage the full hand mudra.

Practice

Form your dominant hand into Doe Seal (*mrigi mudra*) by bringing your hand to your nose (being careful to keep your head turned straight ahead and not rotating toward the hand), and blocking your right nostril with your thumb (or your ring finger if you're left-handed). Gheranda says to inhale for 16 counts, but that's way too extreme; start with a count of 4 or 5 on both the inhalations and exhalations, and don't perform any internal retention yet. Now block your left nostril and exhale through the right, pause briefly, and inhale through your right. Finally block the right nostril and open and exhale through the left. This is one cycle; repeat five to ten times.

As you gain experience with *sahita,* you can begin to regularize the inhalations and exhalations. First use the same count for both, gradually lengthening it to a comfortable number, then extend the count of the exhalation to twice that of the inhalation. We'll work on retention soon, and this can be added to the mix at some point in the future.

Traditional Benefit

The benefits of *sahita pramayama* seem too good to be true. It grants us the ability to move through space (*kha*); to destroy disease; to awaken *shakti* and quiet the mind; and best of all, to be happy (*sukha*).

SECTION 2: FOUR PRANAYAMAS

The first breath in this section, *ujjayi,* can be practiced either reclining or sitting, though I'll only describe the latter. *Surya bhedana* and *bhramari* are best performed sitting up, and *shitali* can be done during asana practice. Assume a comfortable seat for the first three breaths.

CONQUEROR (UJJAYI)

> JAYA • conquering, winning; triumph, being victorious (in battle, in playing with dice, or in a lawsuit); victory over or restraint of the senses

Conqueror is one of the foundation breaths of modern *pranayama,* at least in the Iyengar approach. Its early form in the *Hatha-Yoga-Pradipika* is slightly different than its modern incarnation. According to Svatmarama, the inhalation is made through both nostrils, as it is today, but the exhalation is made only through the left nostril, the right being blocked with a fingertip. Three hundred and fifty years later, Gheranda described the breath (or the inhalation; he said nothing about the exhalation) much as we practice it today.

Practice

Gheranda is the soul of brevity: inhale and retain the breath for as "long as comfortable," applying Net-Bearing Bond. Svatmarama notes that Conqueror can be practiced while walking (*Hatha-Yoga-Pradipika* 2.53), which might make an interesting breathing experiment while you're out hiking in the park.

Following are a pair of techniques to work with Conqueror, *ajapa mantra* and ratio breathing. Retention (*kumbhaka*) will be covered in Section 3.

UNWHISPERED MANTRA (AJAPA MANTRA)

JAPA · muttering, whispering; muttering prayers, repeating passages from scripture, charms, or names of deities in a murmuring tone

MANTRA · "instrument of thought" [i.e., *man,* "to think" and *tra,* "instrument"]; speech, sacred text or speech, a prayer or song of praise; a Vedic hymn or sacrificial formula; a mystical verse or magical formula (sometimes personified), incantation, charm, spell (especially in modern times employed by the Shaktas to acquire superhuman powers; there is thought to be 70 million primary mantras and innumerable secondary ones

The yogis say the "unwhispered" (*ajapa*) mantra is spoken with every breath we breathe, 21,600 times a day (15 times a minute).

Practice

Inhale through your nose, open your mouth wide, and breathe out with a long *ha* sound. Ideally, this mouthed exhalation will pass naturally over the back of your throat. Repeat three or four times. Close your mouth and both inhale and exhale through your nose, but as you did with the mouthed exhalation, direct the breath over the back of your throat.

Now close your eyes and breathe through your nose for a few minutes with the breath passing over the back of your throat. Listen carefully to the sound. As much as possible, make that sound smooth and even, so it sounds pretty much the same from start to finish.

Traditional Benefit

None are listed in our three main sourcebooks, but according to modern sources, directing the breath over the back of the throat slows its normal speed and amplifies its natural sound, which is useful in monitoring its flow.

LITTLE LAMP: HAMSA

HAMSA · goose, gander, swan, flamingo (or other aquatic bird, considered as a bird of passage, sometimes a mere poetical or mythical bird); the soul or spirit (typified by the pure white color of a goose or swan, and migratory like a goose); sometimes the Universal Soul or Supreme Spirit

The unwhispered mantra is also known as the HAMSA mantra because, as Gheranda relates, the breath exhales with the sound *ham* and inhales with the sound *sa.* The HAMSA, Heinrich Zimmer writes, "symbolizes the divine essence . . . embodied in, and abiding with, the individual, yet . . . forever free from, and unconcerned with, the events of individual life."[1] By constantly listening to the "humming" of this name in the breath, the yogi discovers this "inner presence" in herself.

RATIO BREATHING

Ratio breathing (a modern term) is based on Gheranda's description of both *nadi shuddhi* and *sahita pranayama* (see, for example, *Gheranda-Samhita* 5.49ff.). The traditional ratio is expressed as 1:4:2(:1); that is, for every 1 count of inhalation, there are 4 counts of internal retention, 2 counts of exhalation, and though not mentioned by Gheranda, usually 1 count of external retention. For this exercise, we'll work only with inhalation and exhalation, and leave retention for the next section.

Practice

To begin this practice, inhale for 3 counts, then exhale for 3 counts. Always establish an equal ratio first. After a few cycles of inhaling and exhaling, lengthen only the exhalation to 4 counts. Take a few more cycles, then if all seems "appropriate," extend the exhalation to 5 counts for a few more cycles. Once this is established comfortably, go to a 6-count exhalation for a few more cycles. If all is still well, lengthen the inhalation to 4 counts, take a few cycles, then lengthen the exhalation to 7 counts. Take a few more cycles, then again add 1 count to the exhalation for a total of 8 counts. At this point, you've reestablished the 1:2 ratio. You can, if all is still well, now lengthen the inhalation to 5 counts and then proceed to increase the exhalation count slowly, one count at a time, to 10 and so on.

Remember not to push yourself beyond a reasonable limit. Find a 1:2 ratio that's *very* comfortable and stay with it for a time. Even Svatmarama cautioned us 650 years ago to work carefully with the breath, as if taming lions and tigers. If done rashly, he said, *pranayama* will "kill" (*hanti*) the breather—no doubt a slight exaggeration, but a point well taken.

Traditional Benefit

Svatmarama says that Conqueror will cure various diseases and increase digestive fire. Gheranda seconds this and adds that mastery of the breath will destroy old age and death.

SUN PIERCING (SURYA BHEDANA)

> SURYA · the sun or its deity (denotes the most concrete of
> the solar gods; he is regarded as one of the original Vedic
> triad, his place being in the sky, while that of Agni is on
> the earth, and that of Indra is in the atmosphere; he moves
> through the sky in a chariot drawn by seven ruddy horses
> or mares)
>
> BHEDANA · piercing, breaking, splitting, cleaving, rending,
> tearing

Surya bhedana is another digital form of *pranayama*, in which the inhalation is taken exclusively through the right nostril (the "sun" side) and the exhalation made exclusively through the left (the "moon" side).

Gheranda is rather more detailed about the practice than Svatmarama. Both agree that the inhaled breath should be held with "great effort" (*bahu yatna*); in fact, Gheranda says to hold it until there's sweat in your "nails" (*nakha*) and "hair" (*kesha*). I'm sure our yogi knew just what he was doing, but I definitely don't recommend following these instructions.

Practice

Form Doe Seal with your dominant hand. Bring the mudra to your nose, block the left nostril, and inhale through the right. Then block the right and slowly exhale through the left. This is the simple pattern for *surya bhedana:* inhale right, exhale left.

Traditional Benefit

Gheranda is more enthusiastic about this breath than Svatmarama. The latter says it cleans the skull and removes various diseases. Gheranda agrees but adds that it also awakens *kundalini.*

Bee (Bhramari)

BHRAMARA · a large black bee

Svatmarama and Gheranda present different versions of this practice, the former's being the more familiar. Gheranda instructs us to go to some quiet place at midnight, plug our ears, retain the breath after an inhalation, and listen for subtle sounds in the right ear. This appears to be equivalent to what Svatmarama calls Nada Yoga (the "Yoga of Subtle Sound"; see chapter 8), or "unstruck sound" (*anahata shabda*). These instructions are followed by a laundry list of sounds the practitioner should listen for — a cricket (*jhilli*), a flute, various drums, a gong, thunder, and a bee among them. It's not clear why Gheranda settled on calling this exercise Bee, since he could just as well have called it Cricket or Kettledrum or Thunder. Was he copying Svatmarama and made a mistake?

Svatmarama's Bee is performed on both the inhalation (quickly, like a male bee) and exhalation (slowly, like a female bee), but the former is much more challenging than the latter. We'll focus on the exhalation only.

Practice

You can close off your ears with your thumbs as in *yoni mudra* (see chapter 6) or, what seems to me more comfortable, insert a foam earplug in each ear. Inhale slowly and silently, then exhale slowly with a beelike humming noise. Listen carefully to the sound you make, ensuring that it's smooth and even from beginning to end; in other words, the sound you make at the start of the exhalation should sound like the one you make near the end of the breath.

Traditional Benefit

This practice bring success (*siddhi*) in *samadi*.

COOLING (SHITALI)

This breath comes in handy on a warm day or after a vigorous practice of Sun Salute (*surya namaskar*).

Practice

Curl your tongue into a tube and stick it out of your mouth. Inhale over your tongue and "swallow" the moisture-cooled breath into your lungs. Perform Net-Bearing Bond and hold the breath in for 5 to 8 seconds; exhale with your head still down. At the end of the exhalation, return your head to an upright position. Repeat several times.

Traditional Benefit

This practice cures indigestion.

SECTION 3: RETENTION (KUMBHAKA)

KUMBHA · jar, pitcher, water pot

Breathing is life, right? And what do we call a state of no breathing? Well, if it lasts more than about six or seven minutes, we usually call it death.

Not surprisingly, the yogis have worked this formula out backward. According to Gheranda, when the body is at rest, the breath leaves it to a distance of "twelve fingers" (*dvadasha anguli;* that is, the width, not the length, of the finger). If we take that literally and use one of my fingers as a standard, then one finger-width equals about three quarters of an inch, so that twelve finger-widths equals 9 inches. Certain activities increase that distance, such as singing, eating, walking, sleeping, sex (which sends the breath out to 27 inches), and exercise. Since the length of a person's life is fixed by karma, there's an expectation that we'll breathe a certain number of times in our life. For example, if, as the yogis claim, we breathe an average of 21,600 times a day, and if our karma schedules us to live for sixty years, we'll have a store of about 473 million breaths—give or take a million—to draw on. But, the argument continues, death isn't very smart, or the number of breaths we're allotted somehow supercedes our given number of years, so if we *slow down* our breathing by about a third to 14,500 times a day, and we still have 473 million breaths to our credit, then we can expect to live another twenty-nine years. Carrying this argument to the extreme, if we don't breathe at all, we'll never draw on our breathing account, and consequently (as strange as it seems), we'll live virtually forever. What Gheranda is saying, in essence, is that breathing is *death*—eventually anyway—rather than eternal life.

If you think all this is reasonable, I've got a bridge I'd like to sell you. But the fact is that *kumbhaka,* retaining the breath in the *kumbha,* or "pot torso," is the central practice in traditional Hatha Yoga. Each of our breaths is suffused with *pranic* energy, which is collected, concentrated, and "heated" in the lower torso through the techniques of *pranayama* and then used to awaken the slumbering *kundalini.* It's important not to follow the traditional instructions here, which generally tell us to hold the breath until little beads of sweat break out on our forehead. This is *hatha,* "force," at its worst. Retention is best learned from a responsible teacher; a book can only take you so far, so our work with this practice will be at a very basic level. If you want to go a bit further but don't have a teacher, then you can look in my two books on *pranayama* for additional instruction.

Although none of our three main sources mention it, there are traditionally two *kumbhakas,* one after the inhalation (called *antara kumbhaka*) and one after the exhalation (*bahya kumbhaka*). In the traditional ratio of 1:4:2:1, the former is four times as long as the inhalation, and the latter equals the inhalation count. However, at this stage of practice, the inner retention count should *never* be longer than the inhalation count. To be clear, our ultimate ratio is 1:1:2:1. Let's start with outer retention, then do inner.

Practice: Outer Retention

In the best of all possible worlds, your early *pranayama* breathing would be practiced while lying supported on a folded blanket, with your chest open to the heavens. But to keep the instruction in this book manageable, you can sit for this practice (and read about reclining breathing, if you like, in my first *pranayama* book). To start, establish an even ratio in Conqueror breath, let's say 3 counts for both inhalations and exhalations (3:0:3:0). When you feel ready, exhale to 3 counts. At the end of the breath, perform Net-Bearing Bond and pause the breath for a count of 3 (3:0:3:3). Net-Bearing here is more of a practice run than any great necessity; stopping your breath for a count of 3 after an exhalation isn't life-threatening in any way. But pay close attention to your brain as you pause for the 3 count, and notice if it tends to quiet down somewhat. Eventually you'll begin to understand why the yogis hold *kumbhaka* in such high regard.

Now you can start increasing the exhalation count as described previously for Conqueror until you reach 3:0:6:3. Ask yourself if all seems well—no irritation, frustration, anger, thoughts of wreaking significant damage on someone or something. If so, then extend your breath to 4:0:8:4 and so on, until you find a reasonably comfortable ratio. At this point in your practice, assuming from my end that you're a relative *pranayama* beginner, your *bahya kumbhaka* is more like a simple breathing pause that takes place naturally at the end of every exhalation than it is a full-blown retention. This is all I'll ask you to do for now, holding the other two bonds in reserve.

Practice: Inner Retention

Please practice inner and outer retention separately for the time being, getting comfortable with the former before you pick up the latter. To start, again establish a 3:0:3:0 ratio, then after every few cycles, add a single *antara kumbhaka* count, starting with 1. Now Net-Bearing is more important: lower your head into the bond as you near the inhalation, hold it during the exhalation, bring your head up and take an everyday breath, then begin again. What I'm saying, just so you don't miss it, is that the inner retentions should be done *every other breath*, with the head up during the nonretention breath. Please don't keep your head down the whole time, which might strain your neck.

Eventually you'll reach 3:3:3:0. At this point, you can again increase the inhalation and exhalation counts, but there's *no pressing need* to do the same with inner retention. Pay close attention to how your brain feels and how the exhalation is initiated. If your brain feels disturbed by the retention or the exhalation comes out with a burst of air, you're holding the breath too long, and you should back off slightly on the length of the retention. Learn to keep the brain quiet and release the breath softly before moving on.

Traditional Benefit

Will retention quiet the brain and prolong life? There's certainly no hard scientific evidence I know of that confirms these claims, but at the same time, there's no hard scientific evidence that disproves them either. At the very least this kind of practice will, if conducted rationally and regularly, make us more efficient breathers, and since breathing is life, even if it doesn't extend our years, we can hope that it will make them happier.

LITTLE LAMP: UNACCOMPANIED RETENTION (KEVALA KUMBHAKA)

KEVALA · exclusively one's own (not common to others); alone, only, mere, sole, one, excluding others; not connected with anything else, isolated, abstract, absolute; simple, pure, uncompounded, unmingled; entire, whole

According to Svatmarama and Anonymous/Gheranda, there are two kinds of *kumbhaka, sahita* and *kevala. Sahita,* as we've seen is accompanied with visualizations and with inhalations and exhalations. It might seem odd to say that this *kumbhaka* includes inhalation and exhalation, but this is considered the "lower" form of retention, what we might call "intentional retention." The other form of *kumbhaka* is *kevala*, which in this context means "unaccompanied," or without inhalation and exhalation. In other words, *sahita kumbhaka* is something we *do*, while *kevala kumbhaka* is something that *happens to* us. It's a spontaneous cessation of the breath that Patanjali calls the "fourth" (*chaturtha*) [breath], when inhalation and exhalation are transcended (*akshepin*; see *Yoga-Sutra* 2.51).

Gheranda, who obviously wasn't holding down a day job, wants us to practice eight times a day, every three hours. Failing that, five times daily, and failing that, three times—at 4:00 A.M., noon, and 8:00 P.M. When we've mastered this breath, he says, the world is pretty much ours. Svatmarama makes the point that *kumbhaka* stirs *kundalini* to life, and so success is ours.

SECTION 4: MISCELLANEOUS PRANAYAMAS

I've relegated these practices to the bench in this book because, in my opinion, they're either too obscure (for example, Swooning and Floating) or too difficult to learn from a book (common to *Hatha-Yoga-Pradipika* and *Gheranda-Samhita*).

BELLOWS (BHASTRIKA)

BHASTRA · a bellows or large hide with valves and a clay nozzle

Bellows is a vigorous form of Skull Brightening (see chapter 3). While the latter includes only an active exhalation, Bellows includes both an active inhalation and an active exhalation.

Practice

Each session of traditional Bellows consists of three rounds of 20 breaths each, each round concluding with breath retention. This breath is more vigorous than in Skull Brightening and is best learned from an experienced teacher.

Traditional Benefit

This practice supports daily health.

SWOONING (MURCHCHHA)

MURCHCHHA · fainting, swooning

Swooning, or Fainting, is an unfortunate name for this exercise; of course, the original authors never imagined they would be translated into English with this particular word. The implication of both "swoon" and "faint" suggests the practitioner will end up falling over in an unconscious heap. This doesn't, however, seem to be the case; rather, it appears that the exercise is a form of *shambhavi mudra*.

Practice

Comfortably (*sukha*) hold the breath and, withdrawing consciousness from all thoughts and joining it with the self, fix the consciousness at the middle of the forehead (*bhru*).

Traditional Benefit

The practitioner feels blissful (*ananda*).

SIT [SOUND] MAKING (SITKARA)

SIT · onomatopoeic imitation of the sound of breath
KARA · making

This practice is often used as a substitute for *shitali*. Apparently some percentage of the population can't form the rolled-up tongue needed for Cooling breath. *Sitkari*, literally "making the sound *sit*," creates a similar cooling effect.

Practice

Spread your lips and set your teeth lightly. Inhale between your teeth, then follow the postinhalation directions for Cooling breath.

Traditional Benefit

This practice cures indigestion.

FLOATING

> *PLAVA* · swimming, floating

Have you ever tried a flotation tank, also called a sensory deprivation tank, in which a person floats in body-temperature water in silent darkness. It's an experience you'll want to have at least once in your life. In a way, it cancels out the pull of gravity and to some extent frees the breathing apparatus from its customary restrictions. You can get an idea of what it's like by breathing while lying in a warm bath.

Practice

Swallow air (yes, you can do this if you try—but don't) until your stomach is bloated, then go float in water.

Traditional Benefit

Floating in water like a lotus seems to cause happiness.

TURN OUT THE LIGHT

> *SATTVA* · being, existence, entity, reality; true essence, nature, disposition of mind; vital breath, life, consciousness, strength of character, strength, energy, resolution, courage, self-command, good sense, wisdom, magnanimity; the quality of purity or goodness
>
> *DHI* · thought, especially religious thought, reflection, meditation, devotion, prayer (holy thoughts personified); understanding, intelligence, wisdom, knowledge; mind, disposition, intention, design

Once again, it's important to keep in mind that Hatha Yoga is more than just a physical practice. Svatmarama makes the point, often overlooked, that *pranayama* requires not only a pure physical body, but a pure consciousness as well. He advises us to practice with a *sattvic dhi*. My source translators usually leave *sattva* untranslated, no doubt exasperated by the bewildering possibilities (as you can see in the preceding translation). *Dhi* is typically rendered as "mind," but here again the translators have settled for the lowest common denominator. What Svatmarama is calling for in *pranayama* is a mind suffused with "strength, energy, resolution, courage, self-command, good sense, wisdom, magnanimity, and purity or goodness."

8

MEDITATION

vidyapratitih svagurupratitir atma pratitir manasah prabodhah
dine dine yasya bhavetsa yogi sushobhanabhyasamupaiti sadyah

If you have "faith" (*pratiti,* "clear apprehension or insight
into anything, complete understanding or ascertainment,
conviction; confidence, faith, belief; trust, credit; delight")
in your wisdom, your teacher, and in your own self,
then very quickly you'll establish a practice that's
most "splendid" (*sobhanna,* "brilliant, beautiful;
excellent, glorious, magnificent, distinguished;
propitious, auspicious; virtuous, moral;
correct, right").

—A loose translation of
Gheranda-Samhita 7.2

AT MY YOGA SCHOOL in Oakland, we publicize upcoming events
with fliers sporting catchy titles across the top of the page. Recently we
put one out for a Yoga and Meditation workshop that, after a few days,
struck me as very odd. Yoga *and* meditation makes it seem like the latter
is something different than the former, and I guess it is in the twenty-first
century West. Our idea of yoga is mostly asana; we yoga people leave
the meditation up to the Buddhists, who we then look at askance because their sitting posture is generally what we consider to be deplor-
able. But go back far enough and you'll find that meditation rounds off
the practice of every one of the old yoga books. Far from being an "and,"

meditation was an essential "is" of the overall practice in all three of my sourcebooks; in fact, in the *Shiva-Samhita*, the final chapter on meditation is by far the longest of the book's five chapters, comprising 40 percent of its verses.

MEDITATION PRACTICE OVERVIEW

What is Hatha Yoga meditation? Gheranda lists six forms of meditation that make up what he calls Raja Yoga (Royal Union-Method):

Shiva's Seal (*shambhavi mudra*), which we'll cover in Section 3 of this chapter

Bee breath (*bhramari pranayama*), covered in chapter 7

Space-Walking Seal (*khechari mudra*), covered in chapter 6

Womb Seal (*yoni mudra*)

Devotional Yoga (*bhakti yoga*), which Gheranda describes as a "heart" visualization of your "beloved" (*ishta*, "wished, desired; liked; reverenced, respected; sacrificed, worshiped with sacrifices") deity

Swooning (*murchchha*), covered in chapter 7

As you can see, we've already covered three of these meditations, and another will be described in this chapter. The other two I don't find particularly useful, so I've chosen three simple meditations from the *Shiva-Samhita* that I do find engaging: one involves an imaginative focus on a point inside the head; another involves an inside-the-head visualization of the moon; and the third entails a highly imaginative focus on a point *outside* the head. I've also included a meditation from the *Hatha-Yoga-Pradipika* that, while not especially accessible, almost has to be included here because of the importance Svatmarama gives it.

Section 1: Head Meditation 1

Meditation on the Back of the Head (*shira pashcha*) (*Shiva-Samhita* 5.71)

Section 2: Head Meditation 2

Meditation on the Top of the Head ("Brahma Hole," *brahma randhra*) (*Shiva-Samhita* 5.178–181)

Interior Moon (*chandra*) (*Shiva-Samhita* 5.182–90)
Variation: Kailash (*Shiva-Samhita* 5.191–94)
Section 3: Open-Eye Meditation
Shiva's Seal (Shambhavi Mudra; *Hatha-Yoga-Pradipika* 4.35–41;
Gheranda-Samhita 3.53-56)
Little Lamp: The Eye of Shiva (Rudra Aksha; *Gheranda-Samhita*
5.62–64)
Section 4: Bonus Practice: Nada Yoga (*Hatha-Yoga-Pradipika*
4.64–114)

For each practice that follows, assume a comfortable but erect sitting pose, either on the floor (on a support and/or against a wall to support the back torso if needed) or on a chair. Lay your hands in your lap or on your knees, and close your eyes. When you first start these practices, stay for about a minute—no, that's not a misprint, a minute. All of these exercises ask you to concentrate and hold your awareness at a specific point, and until you have some practice under your belt (or unless you're already an experienced meditator), it'll take you some time to maintain a steady connection. When you feel comfortably established at a minute, add 15 seconds and practice for 75 seconds until you again feel comfortable. Continue in this way until you reach 5 minutes, which may take several weeks or months. At this point, you may settle in or continue on to longer sittings—increasing your time incrementally—as your schedule allows.

SECTION 1: HEAD MEDITATION 1

MEDITATION ON THE BACK OF THE HEAD (SHIRA PASHCHA)

SHIRA · head
PASHCHA · back

If I asked you to draw a picture of yourself, what would you do? Without much thought, I believe most people would draw themselves from the front, face on, which is, of course, how most people picture themselves. However, it's possible to draw yourself from many different angles and perspectives—from the side, for example, or looking down on the top of your head, or from the back. Indeed, while we all have a fairly clear picture of what we look like from the front, since we can see much of that side directly or indirectly in a mirror, we don't have a very good idea of what our back side looks like at all, especially the back of our head.

What would happen if we looked at ourselves, figuratively speaking, from the back of our head? My students report various reactions with such a meditation, from a noncommittal "eh . . ." to an enthusiastic account of new insights and inspirations. I'm somewhere between these two extremes; I enjoy the challenge of maintaining this perspective—I'm so unaccustomed to doing it that my consciousness is just "aching" to move forward—and, if I'm successful, it gives me a sense of calm that's quite enjoyable.

Practice

The *Shiva-Samhita* devotes one succinct line to this practice: "meditate on the back of your head." Here's how I've interpreted this instruction. You can either sit in a comfortable yoga seat or lie on your back, perhaps with your torso propped up on a folded blanket. Imagine withdrawing the awareness or consciousness pervading your body to a point, like a massive star whose matter has collapsed into a black hole the size of a marble. Then position this point at the back of your head, just where it joins the back of your neck, and hold it there.

At first you may find this seemingly simple exercise unusually and frustratingly difficult. Persist. Eventually your consciousness marble will accept what you're asking it to do and stay put—for the most part. Hold this point in place for a while, depending on the time available for practice, anywhere from 5 to 15 minutes. Then allow the point to expand, and from the back of your head, allow your awareness to seep back into the rest of your body.

Traditional Benefit

With customary traditional understatement, the *Shiva-Samhita* promises victory over death.

SECTION 2: HEAD MEDITATION 2

MEDITATION ON THE TOP OF THE HEAD (BRAHMA HOLE)

> *RANDHRA* · slit, split, opening, aperture, hole, chasm, fissure, cavity (nine openings are reckoned in the human body, sometimes with a tenth in the skull, as in the fontanel of an infant)

There's an opening at either end of *sushumna nadi*. At the bottom is the Brahma door (*dvara*, "door, gate, passage, entrance; opening, aperture; a way, means, medium"), which is blocked by *kundalini*, but which is also her ingress into the central *nadi* when she's awakened. At the top end is the Brahma "hole" (*randhra*). There are two stages to this exercise, the second being an optional continuation of the first.

Practice, Stage 1

As you did with the previous meditation, gather your awareness to a small point, but this time, fix it at the *brahma randhra* at the top of your head.

INTERIOR MOON (CHANDRA, OPTIONAL)

Practice, Stage 2

I've mentioned that we each have an interior "sun" and "moon," the former situated at the solar plexus in the torso and the latter usually placed somewhere in the head. While the previous two meditations involved a simple gathering of awareness to a point inside the skull, this one requires the additional visualization of the full "moon" at the cranial vault, the top inside of the skull.

So, just inside the top of the head, visualize the brilliant white light of the full moon. Anonymous/Shiva completes this picture by having this imaginary moonlight shining down on a "sea of milk" that fills the interior of the skull.

Traditional Benefit

These two meditations send Anonymous/Shiva into paroxysms of ecstasy. Even if I toned down what he has to say, it would sound extreme. Let's just say they have a salubrious effect on consciousness, and that regular practice brings us closer to our authentic self.

LITTLE LAMP: *SHIVA-SAMHITA* 5.180

There's a curious contradiction between my source translations in verse 5.180. The most recent one, published in 2007, reproduces the last part of the second line of the verse as, "I [Shiva] shall give him knowledge and quickly make him cross to the other side." However, the other two translations, published in 1914 and 1998, include a word in that line not shown in the more recent translation: *bhuta,* the "world." So the rendering is completely different (from the 1998 volume): "By giving the spiritual knowledge, he delivers liberation to other people as well." Of course, we'd like to think the latter translation is the correct one; spreading the good word is always preferable to keeping it secret. But this dissemination seems to be contradicted in the very next verse when Shiva says, "This knowledge of the *brahma randhra* given by me should be kept secret with great care." We'll assume that the newest translation is most definitive, but that the older ones, despite possibly being corrupt, have the more appealing idea about sharing our insights and inspirations.

VARIATION: KAILASH (SHIVA-SAMHITA)

The first two meditations focused on points inside the skull, and the third added a visualization of the interior moon. But the yogis also make use of imaginary points outside the body. For example, two of these points in traditional Hatha Yoga are located about a foot in front of the nose and about a foot above the crown. They're called the end-of-twelve (*dvadashanta*) because each is situated about twelve finger-widths (about 12 inches) away from the body.

Kailasha ("crystalline, icy," from *kelas*, "crystal") is the name of an actual mountain in the Tibetan Himalayas, honored as the home of Shiva, and so a popular pilgrimage site. Rather than going through all the trouble of traveling to this site, the yogis simply imagine it situated above the head, although Anonymous/Shiva doesn't provide us with any visual elements. Since the name comes from "crystal," I imagine it as a shining (*las*) crystal ball.

Practice

You can make an imaginary pilgrimage to the holy mountain. It's relatively easy to find a spot inside your head, but somewhat more challenging to locate one about a foot outside it. Just remember that this isn't rocket science, and the spot doesn't really have to be exactly a foot. It's simply somewhere "up there," a bit above your crown.

SECTION 3: OPEN-EYE MEDITATION

SHIVA'S SEAL
(SHAMBHAVI MUDRA)

> **SHAMBHU** · being or existing for happiness or welfare, granting or causing happiness, beneficent, benevolent, helpful, kind; another name for Shiva

Shambhu is another name for Shiva, so this exercise is called Shiva's Seal. To some it might seem odd to include a seal in the meditation section, and I might be offending the staunchest traditionalists. But it seems to me that this exercise, like all typical meditations, "seals" awareness on a focal point and prevents it from wandering off. The seal involves a kind of paradox, which is the instruction to do two opposite things at the same time. Normally when we meditate, we're asked to "go inside," to turn our awareness away from the outside world and focus on the inner, to be conscious of consciousness itself. But this inevitably sets up a duality between what we imagine is "out there" and what's "in here." If, as Gheranda says, the "entire universe" (*sarva jagat*) is Vishnu, then what's out there should ultimately be included in our meditation. This is exactly what *shambhavi mudra* does.

Trataka (see chapter 3) is frequently suggested as a preparation for this exercise.

LITTLE LAMP: THE EYE OF SHIVA (RUDRA AKSHA)

RUDRA · crying, howling, roaring; dreadful, terrific, terrible, horrible; (cap.) early name for Shiva

AKSHA · eye

Another possible preparation for *shambhavi mudra* is the Eye of Shiva, which teaches us the preliminary step of concentrating our awareness at the bridge of the nose.

Practice

Although he doesn't cite its exact location, it's safe to assume, from the iconography of the Hatha tradition, that Anonymous/Shiva locates the Shiva eye at the bridge of the nose. He instructs us to visualize a "hole" (*vivara*, "fissure, chasm, slit, cleft, hollow, vacuity") there, from which will flash a light as bright as lightning (*vidyut*).

Svatmarama is slightly more detailed about this practice than Gheranda. First, focus on a point "inside" the body. A number of points are possible — any of the chakras along the spine, for instance — but I recommend the spot behind the bridge of the nose, variously known as Shiva's Place (*shiva sthana*), the command wheel (*ajna chakra*), and the eye of gnosis (*jnana cakshus* or *netra*).

As you did with the Meditation on the Back of the Head, gather your awareness to a point, but this time, position it at the *shiva sthana* and fix it there steadily. When you feel ready, open your eyes no more than halfway, and "look out" at whatever's in front of you but "don't see." By "look," I mean to simply accept whatever picture reaches your eyes without "seeing" or "naming" it. Try not to move your eyes or even blink.

Traditional Benefit

Practicing this meditation destroys sins, so that even a wicked (*dura-cara*) person can reach the highest state (*parama pada*). Shiva's Seal is also supposed to quiet the mind. Mark Dyczkowski explains it as follows:

> Although the adept's attention [may be] outwardly directed, he enjoys contemplative absorption through the introverted aspect of *Kramamudra* [i.e., another name for Shambhavi]. Initially he turns inward from the outside world and [then] from within [himself] he exits into the outer world under the influence of his absorption. Thus the sequence (*krama*) in this attitude (*mudra*) [ranges through] both inner and outer.[1]

LITTLE LAMP: WHY NOT BLINK?

On average, we blink twenty times each minute, the average time for each blink being about a quarter second. That means for every waking minute, our eyes are closed for about five seconds, and for every hour, they're closed for five minutes. We blink faster when we're excited, anxious, or under emotional stress, so it seems that the traditional instruction not to blink was meant, at least in part, to quiet the mind. It's also probable that the injunction "no blinking" was intended to maintain a continuous connection between subject and object, so that the simultaneous meditation on the inner and outer points of focus would not be interrupted.

SECTION 4: BONUS PRACTICE—
NADA YOGA

NAD · to make resound or vibrate; to make resonant

Nada Yoga is usually taught today with music, or "audible sound," although to say that seems redundant. After all, isn't all sound audible? But this is the yoga world we're visiting, which is through the looking glass and down the rabbit hole, where inaudible or "unstruck" (*anahata*) sound is a fact of life. Coincidentally, as I sit here typing at my desk, there are fire engines hurrying by, sirens blaring, a few streets over — a full-throated example of audible sound. But the unstruck sound is internal music, coming not from the outside and streaming in, but emanating from "inside" and filling the head with what's described as "spotless, stainless, clean, pure, shining" (*amala*) sound. Though it seems esoteric to us, Svatmarama says, somewhat disparagingly, that the interesting thing about Nada Yoga is that it's appropriate even for "ignorant" (*abodha*) people, and that of 10.25 million ways of achieving ultimate self-understanding, concentration on the *nada* is the best.

I myself have never heard any sound I would characterize as subtle, but that doesn't mean this practice has no value. I'm offering it as a bonus or experiment; at the very least, it will help improve your ability to focus on your own internal processes.

Preliminary

Svatmarama is very specific about the setup for listening to the *nada*. He wants us to sit in Freedom Pose (see chapter 5), and block our eyes, ears, nose (partially, I assume), and mouth with our fingertips, a seal he calls *shambhavi mudra* (Shiva's Seal; not to be confused with Gheranda's Shambhavi, which has the same name but is a different exercise altogether), which nowadays is called *shanmukhi mudra* (see *Light on Yoga* #106). This is all well and good, but holding your hands up for the time it may take to contact the *nada* might be tiring and a distraction, so I recommend using a pair of foam plugs to close your ears and keeping your eyes closed, perhaps with an Ace bandage as a blindfold, and just resting your hands in your lap.

Practice

It's not clear to me exactly where the sound is heard, and maybe I'm being too rational about the whole experiment. Initially we're told to listen for the sound in the right ear, but in the next breath, Svatmarama says the sound is heard in the "pure" (*shuddha*) *sushumna nadi*. It's possible that the source of the sound in the body is the *nadi*, which acts something like a radio receiver, picking up the emanations of the sound from its ultimate source in the Absolute, and that the sound is physically heard in the ear.

Svatmarama uses an interesting word for the way in which we should listen: *ekadhi*. My translators render this as "single-mindedly," or with a "collected" or "concentrated mind," but the word breaks down literally as "one" (*eka*) "thought, especially a religious thought, reflection, meditation, devotion, prayer" (*dhi*). So while these renderings aren't incorrect, they don't relay the all-important qualification that the concentrated listening should be done not only as a meditation, but also as a kind of devotional prayer.

What we'll hear, if we're fortunate, is a series of increasingly subtle sounds. I assume that since these sounds are all unstruck (that is, not created in the usual way, by striking two things together), Svatmarama's list of sounds heard is merely a "struck" approximation, and we're not actually hearing drums or flutes or bells or, mysteriously, a "cloud" (*megha*). As these sounds climb the subtle ladder back to their source in "highest" *brahman*, the mind is gradually absorbed and silenced, until the limited self is dissolved and the yogi is liberated (*mukta*) or realizes his true self, which amounts to the same thing.

Benefit

The benefits of Nada Yoga are numerous and impressive. In no particular order, the yogi will get a divine body (*divya deha*); be wise; be united with the gods; receive powers (*siddhis*); and be free of deficiencies (*dosha*), misery (*duhkha*), old age (*jara*), and sickness (*vyadhi*).

LITTLE LAMP: SOUND

The yogis distinguish between four states (*bhava*) of sound, though it might be more accurate to say that all sound, whether random or organized, broadcasts from the same "soundless" source in three increasingly "soundful" extensions. The creation of the world exactly parallels the uttering of a word. The former evolves from transcendent unity to incarnate diversity, a process that involves a step-by-step splitting off of objects (or the known) from the subject (or the knower);

similarly, the word, as it issues from the depths of our subconscious, first into thought and then in speech, becomes an object for the subject or speaker.

The source of sound is called the "supreme sound" or "supreme voice" (*para vach*). Like the blank screen in a movie theater, which itself remains unchanged while the pictures dance across it, *para vach* is sound's transcendent, perfectly quiescent background. At this stage, there's no differentiation into subject and object, and so no world and nothing to say. In *para vach,* the world/word exists only in potential.

The first faint stirring of *para vach*'s world/word-building impulse gives rise to the second state, called "visible sound" (*pashyanti shabda*). This unusual phrase needs some explanation, since *pashyanti* is still located in the wholly subjective sphere and certainly can be neither seen by the physical eye nor heard by the physical ear. The root of this word means, in its simplest and most literal sense, "to see, look at, observe." Here though, it's used in a more specific sense to mean "to see with the spiritual eye, to have insight or discernment." In this stage, we have an intuitive "vision" of the world to come and what we want to say about it, but there's still no distinct separation between self and other. We've only an intense desire to be a separate self and to express that self in and through the other, the world of objects.

The third state is called the "middle sound" (*madhyama shabda*) simply because of its location in the middle of the second and fourth states, between the sheer possibility of the world/word and the world/word's palpable inception and sounding out. Middle sound is also known as "hidden speech," because it's associated with ideation and reason. At this stage, we're finally in familiar territory. The world is now assuming a shape, with a thoughtful difference between self and other, though it's not until the fourth state that we actually speak our minds.

This last state is called, appropriately enough, "corporeal sound" (*vaikhara shabda*)—sound that at last has a "body" as the world/word. Several interesting explanations have been offered for the Sanskrit word *vaikhari*; for instance, it's said to be what is in that which is most solid (*vikhara*), the body, or that which certainly (*vai*) enters (*ri*) the space (*kha*) of the ear. Corporeal sound, whether random or organized, is the sound of Western science and the everyday world, including human speech (*vach*).

This graduated emergence of everyday sound from its soundless source has been compared to the process of human birth, in which the child first exists only as an abstraction in the loving thoughts of its parents, then as a fertilized egg, then as a fetus, and finally as a neonate. Like every living creature, every sound is rooted in and infused with some quality of its "parent," *shabda brahman*. Every sound we make, then, is a "child" of ours and thus a little world-creation.

TURN OUT THE LIGHT

After reading and studying these sourcebooks for many years, I'm still not sure I understand what's going on. There are at least three hurdles we Westerners have to clear when reading one of the old books. First, they were never meant to be instructional manuals for a mass audience; rather, they were intended as mostly brief outlines of the school's system for a small coterie of initiates — *Cliff's Notes* for *sadhus* — who needed only a summary of the teachings with which they were already more or less familiar. So the instructions are, to be generous, the soul of brevity, omitting what we would consider essential details that leave noninitiates like us in the dark about exactly what's being taught and how the practice should be carried out. Next, the authors often wrote about experiences that are, to a greater or lesser extent, ineffable — like subtle channels and centers, strange juices and unstruck sounds — and so turned to images and metaphors that were rich with meaning for their in-the-know contemporaries but are all too often lost on a twenty-first-century Western reader. Finally, it's not uncommon for the book to be the product of more than one author, even though only one name is on what passes for a title page. The original document is buried under layers of emendations, not infrequently made by an author or authors not especially concerned with consistency. So the teaching, already detail-challenged, can be rife with contradictions and confusions.

Still these men were (mostly) onto something, though it's hard to say exactly what. I'm sometimes almost convinced that the outward physical practice, like the alchemists' lead-into-gold cover story, is all a code for an exquisitely subtle internal practice involving imaginative seats and winds and wheels, all focused on a dormant power each of us harbors in the darkest place of our psyche — the awakening of which turns leaden, mundane lives into spiritual gold. So the old books, seeming to be rather dry instructional manuals on the outside, are actually more like long, secret poems. If we can interpret them accurately (and that's a big *if*), they'll take us first to the depths of our soul, then along the Yellow Brick Road to the glittering Emerald City at its heights.

But many of the old practices, as I've already said, are gone forever, at least to the way we practice Hatha in the West. Many but not all. We have to see for ourselves what gems are hidden in the deceptively simple exercises the old yogis practiced and try to make sense of their purported miraculous results. No disease! Live forever! Reverse the aging process (my personal favorite since I passed my sixtieth birthday)! This book is a first step, by which I hope to encourage you to go and hunt, like you searched for Easter eggs as a kid, for the treasures possibly buried in the pages of wisdom we've blessedly inherited from the old yogis. We're all engaged in the great enterprise of Western Hatha Yoga, now just getting to its wobbly feet like a baby taking its first steps.

Finally we can ask: when we "grow up," where are we heading? Traditional Hatha Yoga has three goals we can adapt and make our own. First, we all know that liberation from our mistaken exclusive identification with the small self or ego, and the resulting release from existential sorrow, is the primary goal of Hatha Yoga (as it is in virtually all schools of yoga). But it's not the only goal; there are at least two more.

Long life is high on the agenda. Svatmarama, in listing the thirty-two "great accomplished ones" (*maha siddha*) of the Hatha lineage, notes that through the "power" or "efficacy" (*prabhava*) of yoga, these gentlemen have "broken" time's scepter (*kala danda*); in other words, they've conquered death's sovereignty over their lives, and wander through the universe (*brahma anda*, literally "Bhrahma's egg"), though what they're up to out there he doesn't say. I don't know if we can go as far as this, but certainly we can use our practice to improve the quality, both physical and mental, of our daily lives.

Now a third goal involves the supernormal powers (*siddhi*) that reputedly manifest as natural accompaniments to the successful practice of yoga. Most of the third chapter of the *Yoga Sutra* is given over to listing more than thirty of these *vibhutis,* as they're called. When we read this list it seems as if we're entering a fantasy world. But considering the enormous potential for abuse, it's clear why the yogis wanted to keep their knowledge a closely held secret and exclude nonqualified individuals. We remember what happened in the *Star Wars* movies when Obi Wan Kenobi insisted on instructing Anakin Skywalker in the ways of the Jedi Knights, even though he was strongly discouraged from doing so.

The desirability of these powers is open to controversy. Most modern yoga teachers warn us away from them, but David Lorenzen writes in *The Kapalikas and Kalamukhas:*

> In spite of the abundant textual references to various siddhis in classical Yoga texts, many modern Indian scholars, and likeminded Western ones as well, have seized on a single sutra of Patanjali (iii.37) to prove that magical powers were regarded as subsidiary, even a hindrance to final liberation, and consequently not worthy of concentrated pursuit. This attitude may have been operative in Vedantic and Buddhist circles and is now popular among practitioners imbued with the spirit of the Hindu Renaissance, but it was not the view of Patanjali and certainly not the view of medieval exponents of Hatha Yoga.[2]

I certainly don't believe we can manifest such unusual powers. But I do believe that Hatha Yoga, along with helping us to see ourselves more clearly and live more healthfully, can also help us express ourselves more completely in our daily lives and so serve as an effective agent for positive change in the world.

APPENDIX 1

ORIGINAL YOGA PRACTICE GUIDELINES

SVATMARAMA STRESSES the need for practice (1.64–66). Whether we're young (*yuvan*), old (*vriddha*), sick (*vyadhi*), or feeble (*durbala*), he assures us that we'll succeed at yoga with regular practice (*abhyasa*, "repeated or permanent exercise, discipline, use, habit, custom; repeated reading, study; inculcation of a truth conveyed in sacred writings by means of repeating the same word or the same passage; in Yoga philosophy, the effort of the mind to remain in its unmodified condition of purity"). But success isn't possible if we're lazy (*tandrita*) or limit our practice to reading a few books (*shashtra*); dressing like a yogi (Svatmarama uses the word *vesha*, which means "dress, apparel," but also "ornament, assumed appearance, disguising one's self"); or talking the talk without walking the walk. This is the truth (*satya*), he concludes, and about this, there's "no doubt" (*na samshaya*).

THE ORIGINAL YOGA PRACTICE: PRACTICE OVERVIEW

Section 1: The Six Acts
    Skull Cleaning (Kapala Dhauti)
    Skull Brightening (Kapala Bhati)
Section 2: The Thirty-Two-Asana Sequence
    Full Practice
    Short Practice

SECTION 1: THE SIX ACTS

The acts in Sections 3, 4, and 5 in chapter 3 are simply daily or at least regular self-ministrations. The only difference now is that you approach them as yoga practices and perform them with the same care and attention as an asana or *pranayama*.

Practice

The acts in Sections 1 and 2, however, can be done in conjunction with a fuller practice or as individual practices on their own.

SKULL CLEANING (KAPALA DHAUTI)

Skull Cleaning can be done at any time of the day or night, such as when you wake up in the morning or just before you bed down for the night. Aficionados of essential oils can rub the bridge of the nose with their favorite or choose an oil that's appropriate for the time of day or situation. Skull Cleaning is also an excellent preparation for a breathing practice or Corpse Pose.

SKULL BRIGHTENING (KAPALA BHATI)

I like to practice Skull Brightening or Trataka (in Diamond Pose) just before starting my asana practice. It's also possible to use one or both as a preparation for *pranayama*.

SECTION 2: THE THIRTY-TWO-ASANA SEQUENCE

Full Practice

I can't say for sure how long the full practice will take you; it depends largely on how you perform the sequence and how long you hold the poses. But I'd guess that a full-blown practice would take at least an hour, more likely 90 minutes. I think of the full practice as proceeding through three stages.

STAGE 1: PRELIMINARY

It's traditional to begin your practice by acknowledging your teacher or spiritual guide, then setting your intention (*samkalpa*) for the upcoming practice. For this, you might sit in Diamond or Perfected Pose and, depending on your time frame, practice Skull Cleaning and/or Frog Seal for a minute. Then perform Trataka, gazing at the tip of a candle flame, for 3 to 5 minutes. The intention doesn't need to be anything special, for example, just a promise to yourself to stay consciously present during the practice.

STAGE 2: ASANA PRACTICE

After the reclining pair in Section 1 in chapter 5, sit in Diamond and perform one or more rounds of Skull Brightening. The poses beginning with Section 2 and ending with Section 7 in chapter 5 can be performed either unlinked (that is, one after the other with no "bridge" between them) or linked by a Sun Salute–type bridge. It works like this. From Diamond, lean forward, press your hands to the floor (assume this from now on when I write "lean forward"), and step or hop back to Downward-Facing Dog Pose. Swing forward to Plank Pose (unofficially known as *phalaka asana*), lower into Four-Limb Staff Pose (*chaturanga danda asana*), swing up to Upward-Facing Dog Pose, and push back to Downward-Facing Dog. From here, either lower onto your knees and shins, crossing your right ankle under your left, or perform a little bunny hop, landing on your knees and shins (toes turned back) with your ankles already crossed, right under left, and snuggle your perineum down onto your left heel for Lion Pose. After performing this pose on the first side, depending on how vigorous you want your practice to be, you can lean forward, lift your buttocks up, and change the cross of your ankles, or you can step/hop back to Downward-Facing Dog, run through the Sun sequence, and finally kneel down or hop forward again with your ankles reversed. You would do the same for the following poses in Section 2 in chapter 5, without crossing the ankles as you come down from Downward-Facing Dog, but simply setting yourself down with your feet and legs side by side.

Performing the sequence with links can work up quite a sweat. Svatmarama says not to wipe it off, but to rub the "water" (*jala*) born of "fatigue" (*shrama*) into your skin. You might also stop now and again and briefly perform Cooling breath (*shitali pranayama*), either with your tongue curled into a tube or with your lips pursed in Crow Seal.

For Section 3, you would kneel or hop forward from Downward-Facing Dog with your ankles crossed and land lightly on the crossed feet; slide back onto the floor while at the same time stretching your legs straight out in front of your torso; then proceed to Fortunate Pose. After Fortunate, cross your ankles, lean forward, and step or hop back to Downward-Facing Dog. In this way you can run through the original sequence up to Bull Pose; to repeat, from each pose cross your ankles, lean forward, hop back to Dog Pose, and finally from Dog, hop forward, landing with crossed ankles and move into the next pose.

The sequence through Sections 4 and 5 generally proceeds in this fashion: cross your ankles in front of your torso, lean forward, and step or hop back to Downward-Facing Dog. For the backbends in Section 6, after completing each pose, you push back directly into Downward-Facing Dog. From the sequence-ending Downward-Facing Dog, you lower straight down to the floor or do a little hop to Plank Pose and then lower slowly to the floor. For the standing poses in Section 7, try this: from the Downward-Facing Dog that follows the backbend sequence, step or hop forward between your hands and straighten your knees to a standing Forward Bend. From here, raise your torso to standing, then squat to Superior Pose. You can then stand upright again to perform Tree Pose or move from Superior into a standing Forward Bend, step or hop back to Downward-Facing Dog for the bridge sequence, then step or hop forward again for Tree. Finally, complete Sections 8 through 10.

STAGE 3: PRANAYAMA AND MEDITATION

When you've finished Section 10, rest in Corpse Pose (Section 12 in chapter 5) for a few minutes, then proceed to Section 11 in chapter 5 and the *pranayama* practice (see Section 4 in this appendix). If you have the time, perform the Three Greats in preparation for breathing. Be sure to leave enough time for Corpse Pose after breathing. Then you might finish the Original practice with some time in sitting meditation.

You can practice each of these three stages separately or in various combinations at different times of the day. For example, you might start your day with *pranayama,* practice asana in the late afternoon, and finish off the evening with meditation. Alternatively, you could practice asana and *pranayama* in the morning and meditation in the late afternoon or early evening.

Short Practice

Given the fact that many of us work for a living and have families, friends, and outside interests (in other words, a life), our regular practice during the week may necessarily be shorter than our weekend or class-time practice. The Original sequence is divided into sections that can be thought of as "modules," to use an untraditional word. There are various interesting and creative ways to mix and match these sections or add to or subtract from them.

For example, you might practice only Sections 2, 3, and 5 for a forward bend day or Sections 1, 2, 8, and 10 for an inversion day. The sequences aren't carved in stone. You can add in other favorite poses or make less favored ones disappear. My only advice is not to perform Sections 4, 6, 8, or 10 without an adequate warm-up.

Section 3: Mudras

Three Bonds

The Three Bonds are usually practiced during *pranayama*. Until you gain some experience with breathing, continue to work only with Net-Bearing Bond in *pranayama*, practicing Root and Flying-Up Bonds on the side in preparation for the day when you're ready to integrate them into a thriving breathing practice.

Three Greats

I usually practice the Three Greats right before I start my *pranayama* practice. Great Seal is the most useful; the jury is still out on the other two, especially Great Piercer.

Tongue and Lips

These exercises can be done periodically during asana and breathing practice. Most of my students find Frog Seal extremely soothing. I've already mentioned how I use *jihva bandha* as a lead-in to the Lion *garjana*. Crow and Serpent Seals can be used for *shitali pranayama* whenever you feel overheated and want to cool down.

Five Concentrations

The Five Concentrations are very popular with my students. I usually leave out describing the imagery, because typically there's not enough time to do the shapes and colors and mantras and deities justice. But students have a good time pretending to breathe into the different areas of the body, whether I start the breath at the level of the heart or the base of the spine.

Section 4: Pranayama

There's always been some question as to whether or not it's kosher to practice *pranayama* right after an asana practice. Back in the old days, when the yoga dinosaurs still walked the earth, and I was a bright-eyed, bushy-tailed student at the Iyengar Institute in San Francisco, we were strongly discouraged — as only certified Iyengar teachers can do — from practicing *pranayama* after asana. The theory was, if I remember correctly, that after a vigorous asana practice, we're all too tired to give the necessary attention to the breath, and as a result, our breathing practice would be ineffective (and even, it was ominously hinted, dangerous). Because of this, we had to show up at the Institute early in the morning for *pranayama,* wait a half hour, and then proceed to asana.

Now we may well be tired after a three- or four-hour class with a merciless Iyengar instructor, but for most of us not in a teacher training program, our asana practice just isn't that wearying; frankly, if we don't strike while the iron is hot and take care of our *pranayama* practice when the opportunity presents itself after asana, then there's a good chance it won't happen at all. So I say — and I can say this because I'm not Iyengar certified — practice *pranayama* after asana if need be.

Practice

Early on in your practice, it's best to stick pretty much with Conqueror. I use Cooling breath after vigorous asana sequences to, obviously, cool down. Purification of the Channels and Bee breath are excellent preparations for breathing,

Section 5: Meditation

The meditations included in this book are, first off, pieces of evidence I wanted to present to show that such a thing was and is possible in Hatha Yoga. But they're also engaging, and the most engaging of the lot to me is Shiva's Seal, because it's so inclusive, it doesn't divide the inner from the outer and then focus exclusively on the former as so many techniques do.

There are certainly several other simple meditations you can use for your Hatha practice that are just as effective, including witnessing your own breath or the flow of consciousness.

APPENDIX 2

THE LITERATURE OF
HATHA YOGA

PRIMARY SOURCES

Century Composed	*Sanskrit Title* (English Rendering)	Author	English Translation?
10?	*Kaula Jnana Nirnaya* (Discussion of the Knowledge Pertaining to the Kaula Tradition)	Matsyendra**	yes
10–11?	*Siddha Siddhanta Paddhati* (Track of the Doctrine of the Adepts)	Goraksha**	yes*
12	*Amara Natha Samveda* (Dialogue with the Immortal Lord)	Goraksha**	no
12	*Gorakh Bodha* (Illumination of Gorakh)	unknown	yes
12–13	*Goraksha Paddhati* (Goraksha's Tracks; aka *Goraksha Samhita*, Goraksha's Compendium)	Goraksha**	yes
?	*Goraksha Shataka* (Goraksha's Century [of Verses], aka *Jnana Shataka, Jnana Prakasha Shataka*) (fragment of *Goraksha Paddhati*)	Goraksha	yes
(no date)	Yoga Martanda (fragment of *Goraksha Paddhati*)	Goraksha	yes
13	*Ananda Samuccaya* (Mass of Bliss)	unknown	no

263

mid-14	*Hatha Yoga Pradipika* (Light on the Forceful Yoga)	Svatmarama Yogendra	yes
(no date)	*Hatha Pradipika Tika* (Commentary on Light on the Forceful [Yoga]) (commentary on *Hatha Yoga Pradipika*)	Ramananda Tirtha	no
(no date)	*Hatha Pradipika Tipuana* (Gloss on Light on the Forceful [Yoga]) (commentary on *Hatha Yoga Pradipika*)	Umapati	no
13–14	*Yoga Yajnavalkya* (Yajnavalkya's Yoga)	unknown	yes
13–14	*Goraksha Siddhanta Samgraha* (Collection of Goraksha's Doctrines)	unknown	no
14–15	*Brihad Yogi Yajnavalkya Smriti* (Great Codex of the Yogin Yajnavalkya)	Yajnavalkya**	yes*
15	*Goraksha Upanishad* (Secret Doctrine of Goraksha)	unknown	no
16	*Shat Chakra Nirupana* (Investigation of the Six Centers) (sixth chapter of the *Shri Tattva Chintamani*)	Purnananda Svamin	yes
late-16	*Vasishtha Samhita* (Vasishtha's Compendium)	unknown	no
mid-17	*Hatha Ratna Avali* (String of Jewels on Hatha [Yoga])	Shrinivasa Bhatta	yes
late-17	*Gheranda Samhita* (Gheranda's Compendium)	unknown	yes
late-17	*Shiva Samhita* (Shiva's Compendium)	unknown	yes
18	*Goraksha Siddhanta Samgraha* (Collection of Goraksha's Doctrines)	unknown	no
18	*Hatha Sanketa Candrika* (Moonlight on the Conventions of Hatha [Yoga])	Sundara Deva	yes*
18	*Hatha Tattva Kaumudi* (Moonlight on the Principles of Hatha [Yoga])	Sundara Deva	yes

18?	*Goraksha Vacana Samgraha* (Collection of Goraksha)	unknown	no
late-18	*Yoga Karnika* (Ear Ornament of Yoga)	Aghorananda	no
late-18	*Yoga Chintamani* (Thought Gem of Yoga)	Shivananda Sarasvati	yes*
mid-19	*Yoga Taranga* (Wave of Yoga)	Deva Tirtha Svamin	yes*
late-19	*Jyotsna* (Moonlight) (on the *Hatha Yoga Pradipika*)	Brahmananda (also authored *Shat Chara Pradipika* and *Shakta Ananda Tarangani*)	yes*
(no date)	*Amanaska Yoga* (Transminded Yoga)	Ishvara Vamadeva	yes
(no date)	*Amaraugha Prabodha* (Awakening to the Immortal Flood)	Goraksha**	no
(no date)	*Amaraugha Shasana* (Instruction on the Immortal Flood)	Goraksha	no
(no date)	*Ananta Vakya* (Infinite Speech)	Carpata**	no
(no date)	*Carpata Shataka* (Carpata's Century [of Verses])	Carpata**	no
(no date)	*Goraksha Shataka Tika* (Commentary on Goraksha's Century) (commentary on *Carpata Shataka*)	Shankar*	no
(no date)	*Goraksha Shataka Tippana* (Gloss on Goraksha's Century) (commentary on *Carpata Shataka*)	Mathura Shukla	no
(no date)	*Carpata Manjari* (Carpata's Flower-Ornament) (commentary on *Carpata Shataka*)	Carpata**	no
(no date)	*Goraksha Bhujanga* (Goraksha's Serpent)	Lakshmidhara	no

(no date)	*Goraksha Kalpa* (Goraksha's Precepts)	Goraksha**	no
(no date)	*Goraksha Vijaya* (Goraksha's Victory)	Goraksha	no
(no date)	*Hatha Yoga Dhiraya*	Shiva**	no
(no date)	*Hatha Yoga Dhiraya Tika* (Gloss on Intelligence of Hatha Yoga) (commentary on *Hatha Yoga Dhiraya*)	Ramananda Tirtha	no
(no date)	*Hatha Yoga Viveka* (Discrimination of Hatha Yoga)	Isvara Vamadeva	no
(no date)	*Jnana Amrita* (Immortal Nectar of Wisdom)	Goraksha**	no
(no date)	*Jnana Amrita Tippana* (Commentary on Immortal Nectar of Wisdom) (commentary on *Jnana Amrita*)	Sadananda	no
(no date)	*Jnana Yoga Khanda* (Fragment on Yoga Gnosis)	unknown	no
(no date)	*Jnana Yoga Khanda Jyotsna* (Moonlight on the Fragment of Yoga Gnosis)	Brahmananda	no
(no date)	*Nava Shakti Shatka* (Six [Stanzas] on the Nine Powers)	Goraksha**	no
(no date)	*Pavana Vijaya Svarodaya* (Victory of the Rising Sound of the Purifying Wind)	unknown	yes*
(no date)	*Shat Karma Samgraha* (Compendium of Right Action)	Cidghanan	yes
(no date)	*Shiva Svarodaya* (Shiva's Rising Sound)	unknown	yes
(no date)	*Uttara Gita* (Later Song of Praise)	unknown	yes*
(no date)	*Yoga Bija* (Seed of Yoga)	Shiva**	yes
(no date)	*Yoga Rahasya* (Yoga Secret)	Nathamuni	no

(no date)	*Yoga Shashtra* (Yoga Teaching)	Dattatreya	no
(no date)	*Yoga Tara Avali* (Sparkling Lines on Yoga)	Shankara**	yes
(no date)	*Yoga Vishaya* (Object of Yoga)	Matsyendra	no

* Summarized in *Encyclopedia of Indian Philosophies*.
** Attributed to this author.

THE YOGA UPANISHADS

These books were written during the fourteenth and fifteenth centuries C.E. and teach a Vedanta-based form of Hatha Yoga.

Book	Found in *Thirty Minor Upanishads*	Summarized in *Encyclopedia of Indian Philosophies*	Available Online
Advaya Taraka (Nondual Deliverer)		X	X
Amrita Bindu (Immortal Point)	X	X	X
Amrita Nada Bindu (Immortal Sound Point)	X		X
Brahma Vidya (Knowledge of the Absolute)		X	X
Darshana (Insight)		X	X
Dhyana Bindu (Meditation Point)	X	X	X
Hamsa (Swan)	X		X
Jabala Darshana (Jabala's Insight)			X
Kshurika (Dagger)		X	X
Maha Vakya (Great Saying)		X	X
Mandala Brahmana (Circle)	X	X	X
Nada Bindu (Sound Point)	X	X	X
Pashu Pata Brahmana (Lord of the Cattle)		X	X

Shandilya (named after sage)	×		×
Tejo Bindu (Radiance Point)	×	×	×
Tri Shikhi Brahmana (Triple Tuft)		×	×
Varaha (Boar)	×		×
Yoga Chuda Mani (Crest Jewel of Yoga)		×	×
Yoga Kundali (Bracelet of Yoga)	×	×	×
Yoga Shikha (Crest of Yoga)			×
Yoga Tattva (Principles of Yoga)	×	×	×

NOTES

Chapter 1. Traditional Hatha Yoga

1. George Weston Briggs, *Gorakhnath and the Kanphata Yogis* (Delhi: Motilal Banarsidass, 1989), 254.
2. Gerald Larson and Ram Shankar Bhattacharya, eds., *Yoga: India's Philosophy of Meditation,* vol. 12 of *Encyclopedia of Indian Philosophies* (Delhi: Motilal Banarsidass, 2008), 503.
3. Margaret Stutley, *The Illustrated Dictionary of Hindu Iconography* (London: Routledge & Kegan Paul, 1985), 120.
4. Swami Vivekananda, *Raja Yoga* (New York: Ramakrishna-Vivekananda Center, 1982), 23.

Chapter 2: Channels and Circuits: Modern Nadis

1. Georg Feuerstein, *The Shambhala Encyclopedia of Yoga* (Boston: Shambhala, 1997), 6.

Chapter 4: Asana through the Ages

1. B. K. S. Iyengar, *The Tree of Yoga* (Boston: Shambhala, 1989), 54–55.
2. Stuart Sovatsky, *Words from the Soul* (Albany, NY: SUNY, 1998), 153–54.
3. Kuvalayananda, *Popular Yoga Asanas,* 33.
4. Quoted in N. E. Sjoman, *The Yoga Tradition of the Mysore Palace* (New Delhi: Abhinav Publications, 1999), 13.
5. K. Narayana Swami Aiyar, trans., "Radiance Point Upanishad," in *Thirty Minor Upanishads* (Delhi: Primal Publications, 2003), 62.

Chapter 5: Gheranda's Thirty-Two Asanas: A Practice Overview

1. B. K. S. Iyengar, *Light on Yoga* (New York: Schocken Books, 1976), 180.
2. Swami Muktibodhananda, commentary, *Asana Pranayama Mudra Bandha* (Munger [Bihar], India: Bihar School of Yoga, 1998), 107.
3. Mabel Elsworth Todd, *The Thinking Body* (Brooklyn, NY: Dance Horizons, 1959), 289–90, 293.
4. Iyengar, *Light on Yoga*, 96.
5. David Gordon White, *Kiss of the Yogini* (Chicago: University of Chicago Press, 2003), 27.
6. Sita Devi Yogendra, *Yoga Physical Education* (Bombay: The Yoga Institute, 1960), 9.
7. Swami Kuvalayananda, *Popular Yoga Asanas* (Rutland, VT: Charles Tuttle, 1971), 67–68.
8. V. K. Jha, Primal Devnath, S. B. Sakhalkar, eds., *Encyclopedia of Traditional Asanas* (Lonavla, India: The Lonavla Yoga Institute, 2006), 110.
9. Theos Bernard, *Hatha Yoga* (New York: Samuel Weiser, 1970), 30.
10. David Gordon White, *The Alchemical Body* (Chicago: University of Chicago Press, 1996), 199.
11. Svatmarama, *The Yoga of Light*, trans. Elsy Becherer, with a commentary by Hans-Ulrich Rieker (New York: Herder and Herder), 127.
12. Heinrich Zimmer, *Philosophies of India* (Princeton, NJ: Princeton University Press, 1971), 57
13. Ibid., 519.
14. Johan Huizinga, *Homo Ludens* (Boston: Beacon Press, 1950), 12.
15. Arthur Avalon, *The Serpent Power* (New York: Dover Publications, 1974), 204.

Chapter 6: Seals and Bonds: Mudras and Bandhas

1. Alain Danielou, *Yoga: Mastering the Secrets of Matter and the Universe* (Rochester, VT: Inner Traditions International, 1991), 53.
2. Theos Bernard, *Hatha Yoga* (New York: Samuel Weiser, 1970), 70.
3. Theos Bernard, *Yoga Gave Me Superior Health* (Natal, South Africa: Essence of Health, 1982), 208.

4. Swami Rama, Rudolph Ballentine, and Alan Hymes, *Science of Breath: A Practical Guide* (Honesdale, PA: Himalayan International Institute, 1979), 122, 124.
5. Swami Satyananda Saraswati, commentary to *Hatha Yoga Pradipika*, by Svatmarama (Munger, India: Bihar School of Yoga, 1998), 320.
6. Kshemaraja, *Shiva Sutras*, trans. Jaideva Singh (Delhi: Motilal Banarsidass, 1990), 101.

Chapter 7: Pranayama

1. Heinrich Zimmer, *Myths and Symbols of Indian Art and Civilization* (Princeton, NJ: Princeton University Press, 1972), 48–49.

Chapter 8: Meditation

1. Mark Dyczkowski, *The Doctrine of Vibration* (Albany, NY: SUNY Press, 1987), 160.
2. David Lorenzen, *The Kapalikas and Kalamukhas* (Berkeley, CA: University of California Press, 1972), 93–94.

GLOSSARY

108 WORDS EVERY HATHA PRACTITIONER SHOULD KNOW

ABHYASA. Diligent practice.

ADHARA. Support, prop.

ADI. Beginning, commencement, primal.

ADVAITA. Nondual (literally "not-two").

AHAMKARA. Literally the "I-maker," ego.

AJAPA. Not pronounced, "whispered."

AMRITA. No-death, deathless.

ANAHATA. Unstruck.

ANJALI. Open hands placed side by side and slightly hollowed (as if by a beggar to receive food; when raised to the forehead, a mark of supplication); reverence, salutation, benediction.

APANA VAYU. Down breath, one of the five major "winds."

ASANA. Seat, place, stool; sitting, sitting down; today it is interpreted as "pose" or "posture."

ATMAN. The self.

AVIDYA. Literally "not-knowing," self-ignorance.

BANDHA. Binding, tying; bond, tie, chain, fetter; damming up (as a river).

BIJA. Seed.

BRAHMA. Holy, sacred, divine; (cap.) the deity of the Hindu trinity that creates the world (see *Shiva, Vishnu*).

BRAHMAN. The Absolute (not to be confused with *Brahma*).

CHAITANYA. Pure consciousness, consciousness without "content."

CHANDRA. Moon.

CHIT. Pure consciousness, consciousness without "content."

CHITTA. Human consciousness, consciousness with "content" (thoughts, feelings, etc.).

DANDA. Staff.

DEVA. Male deity.

DEVI. Female deity.

DHARANA. Holding, bearing, keeping (in remembrance); collection or concentration of the mind (joined with the retention of breath); firmness, steadfastness, righteousness.

DHAUTA. Washed, cleaned, purified.

DHI. Thought, especially a religious thought, reflection, meditation, devotion, prayer.

DHYANA. Meditation.

DIPAKA. Illuminate; a torch; moonlight. This word is a component of *Pradipaka*.

DRISHTI. Gaze.

DUHKHA. Misery, suffering (see *sukha*).

DVARA. Door.

GHATA. Pot; Gheranda's word for the body-mind.

GRANTHI. Knot.

GRIHASTHA. Householder.

GUHYA. Secret, preserved, protected, concealed, hidden.

GURU. "Heavy" one, spiritual preceptor.

HAMSA. Goose, swan.

HATHA. Violence, force; obstinacy, pertinacity; absolute or inevitable necessity.

IDA. Comfort, refreshing; the main *nadi* to the left of *sushumna* (q.v.).

JAPA. Muttering, whispering.

JIVA ATMAN. Living self, a spark of the great self (see *parama atman*).

JNANA. Wisdom.

KAPALA. Skull.

KAPALIKA. Skull Bearer.

KARMA. Act, action, performance.

KAYA. Body.

KEVALA. Alone, sole, pure, simple.

KHA. Cavity, hollow, cave, cavern, aperture.

KUMBHAKA. Potlike; word used for *pranayama* in general and breath retention specifically.

KUNDALINI. Literally "coiled one."

LILA. Play, sport.

MAHA SIDDHA. Great accomplished or perfected one.

MANAS. Human mind.

MANTRA. Instrument of thought, hymn.

MATHA. Yogi's hut.

MERU DANDA. Staff of Meru; refers to the spine.

MITAHARA. Literally "measured eating."

MUDRA. A seal or any instrument used for sealing or stamping.

MUKTA. Liberation, deliverance, beatitude.

MULA. A root (of any plant or tree; also figuratively, the foot or lowest part or bottom of anything); basis, foundation, cause, origin, commencement, beginning.

NADA. Subtle inner sound.

NADI. Tube, pipe; subtle energy channel.

NATHA. Protector, patron, possessor, owner, lord.

NIDRA. Sleep.

PARAMA ATMAN. Great self (see *jiva atman*).

PINGALA. Tawny, reddish brown; the main *nadi* to the right of *sushumna* (q.v.).

PRANA VAYU. Forward breath, one of the five major "winds."

PRANA. Breath of life, breath, respiration, spirit, vitality.

PRASADA. Grace.

RAJA YOGA. Royal Yoga.

RANDHRA. Aperture, hole.

SADHANA. Performance, practice.

SADHU. Straight, right; correct, pure; holy man, saint, sage, seer.

SAKSHIN. Witness.

SAMA. Even, equitable, neutral.

SAMADHI. Putting together, joining or combining with; union.

SAMANA VAYU. Middle breath, one of the five major "winds."

SAMHITA. Compendium.

SAMKALPA. Purpose, intention.

SAMSARA. Literally "wandering through"; the circuit of mundane existence.

SAMSKRITA. Put together, constructed, well or completely formed, perfected. This is the complete form of the word *Sanskrit*.

SHAKTI. Power, ability, strength, might, effort, energy, capability, faculty, skill.

SHASHTRA. Holy scripture.

SHAVA. Corpse.

SHIVA. Auspicious, propitious, gracious, favorable, benign, kind, benevolent, friendly, dear; happy, fortunate; liberation, final emancipation; (cap.) "Auspicious One," the deity of the Hindu trinity that reabsorbs the world (see *Brahma, Vishnu*).

SHODHANA. Cleaning, purifying, refining.

SHUDDHI. Purification.

SIDDHA. Accomplished, fulfilled; perfected, beatified; endowed with supernatural faculties, sacred, holy, divine.

SOMA. Juice, extract.

SUKHA. Ease, happiness, comfort (see *duhkha*).

SURYA. Sun.

SUSHUMNA. Literally "most gracious"; the central *nadi*.

SVAMI. Master, lord. Often spelled *swami*.

TAPAS. Heat; austerity; pain, suffering.

TATTVA. Truth.

UDANA VAYU. Up breath, one of the five major "winds."

VATA. Wind, air.

VAYU. Wind, air; breathing, breath; the wind of the body, a vital air; (cap.) the god of the wind.

VIDYA. Wisdom.

VINYASA. Putting together, connecting.

VISHNU. "All-Pervader," the deity of the Hindu trinity that preserves the world (see *Brahma, Shiva*).

VRITTI. Fluctuation of consciousness.

VYANA VAYU. Distributed breath, one of the five major "winds."

YOGA. Yoking, union-method.

YOGIN. Male practitioner.

YOGINI. Female practitioner.

YONI. Womb, origin.

BIBLIOGRAPHY

Aiyar, K. Narayanasvami, trans. *Thirty Minor Upanishads.* Delhi: Parimal Publications, 2003.

Bandyopadhyay, P. K. *Natha Cult and Mahanad.* Delhi: B. R. Publishing, 1992.

Banerjea, Akshaya. *Philosophy of Gorakhnath.* Delhi: Motilal Banarsidass, 1983.

Briggs, George Weston. *Gorakhnath and the Kanphata Yogis.* Delhi: Motilal Banarsidass, 1989.

Burley, Mikel. *Hatha Yoga: Its Context, Theory and Practice.* Delhi: Motilal Banarsidass, 2000.

De Michelis, Elizabeth. *The History of Modern Yoga.* London: Continuum, 2005.

Feuerstein, Georg. *The Shambhala Encyclopedia of Yoga.* Boston: Shambala, 1997.

———. *The Yoga Tradition.* Prescott, AZ: Hohm Press, 1998.

Larson, Gerald, and Ram Shankar Bhattacharya. *Yoga: India's Philosophy of Meditation.* Vol. 12, *Encyclopedia of Indian Philosophies.* Delhi: Motilal Banarsidass, 2008.

Lorenzen, David. *The Kapalikas and Kalamukhas.* Berkeley, CA: University of California Press, 1972.

Singleton, Mark. *Yoga Body: The Origins of Modern Posture Practice.* Oxford: Oxford University Press, 2010.

Sweigard, Lulu. *Human Movement Potential.* New York: University Press of America, 1974.

Todd, Mabel Elsworth. *The Thinking Body.* New York: Dance Horizons, 1937.

White, David Gordon. *The Alchemical Body.* Chicago: University of Chicago Press, 1996.

———. *Kiss of the Yogini.* Chicago: University of Chicago Press, 2003.

Woodroffe, John. *The Serpent Power.* New York: Dover Publications, 1974.

Zarrilli, Phillip. *When the Body Becomes All Eyes.* New Delhi: Oxford University Press, 1998.

INDEX OF PRACTICES

BOOKS AND AUDIO BY
RICHARD ROSEN

Books

The Yoga of Breath

The Yoga of Breath is a guide to learning the fundamentals of *pranayama* and incorporating them into an existing yoga practice. Rosen's approach is easy to follow with step-by-step descriptions of breath and body awareness exercises accompanied by clear illustrations. The book also covers the history and philosophy of *pranayama,* offers useful practice tips, and teaches readers how to use props to enhance the exercises.

Pranayama beyond the Fundamentals

For serious students of yoga who have an established *pranayama* practice, this book is a follow-up to Rosen's previous book, *The Yoga of Breath*. He picks up where he left off, offering a selection of traditional yogic techniques for those who wish to deepen their practice of *pranayama* and their understanding of the ancient wisdom of yoga. Rosen skillfully puts forward an array of awareness disciplines, breathing practices, *mudras,* and seals, interspersed with anecdotes and quotations from ancient texts.

Audio

The Practice of Pranayama

For thousands of years, yoga practitioners have tapped into the power of *pranayama,* a method of focused breathing, to rejuvenate the body and mind and to bring about spiritual transformation. Here Richard Rosen presents an in-depth program on *pranayama* that is designed for beginners as well as for those with an existing practice who want to build on their experience and refine their technique. On these seven CDs, he offers easy-to-follow, guided breathing instructions and then goes on to lead *pranayama* routines that create an ideal structure for *pranayama* practice at home.